Lupus - Diagnostics and Developments

Edited by Rizwan Ahmad

Published in London, United Kingdom

Lupus - Diagnostics and Developments
http://dx.doi.org/10.5772/intechopen.111266
Edited by Rizwan Ahmad

Contributors
Abdelhamid Naitlho, Abire Allaoui, Alexandru Caraba, Amine Khalfaoui, Deiana Roman, Filipe Soares
Nogueira, Ioannis Gkougkourelas, Ismini Anagnostaki, Konstantia Loga, Konstantinos Zacharis,
Mihaela Nicolin, Mircea Iurciuc, Mohammad Yusuf Hasan, Rita Aniq Filali, Rizwan Ahmad, Rosete
Nogueira, Stela Iurciuc

Notice

Statements and opinions expressed in the chapters are these of the individual contributors and not
necessarily those of the editors or publisher. No responsibility is accepted for the accuracy of
information contained in the published chapters. The publisher assumes no responsibility for any
damage or injury to persons or property arising out of the use of any materials, instructions, methods
or ideas contained in the book.

First published in London, United Kingdom, 2025 by IntechOpen
IntechOpen is the global imprint of INTECHOPEN LIMITED, registered in England and Wales,
registration number: 11086078, 167-169 Great Portland Street, London, W1W 5PF, United Kingdom

For EU product safety concerns: IN TECH d.o.o., Prolaz Marije Krucifikse Kozulić 3, 51000 Rijeka,
Croatia, info@intechopen.com or visit our website at intechopen.com.

British Library Cataloguing-in-Publication Data
A catalogue record for this book is available from the British Library

Lupus - Diagnostics and Developments
Edited by Rizwan Ahmad
p. cm.
Print ISBN 978-0-85466-818-2
Online ISBN 978-0-85466-817-5
eBook (PDF) ISBN 978-0-85466-819-9

If disposing of this product, please recycle the paper responsibly.

We are IntechOpen,
the world's leading publisher of
Open Access books
Built by scientists, for scientists

7,400+
Open access books available

194,000+
International authors and editors

210M+
Downloads

156
Countries delivered to

Our authors are among the

Top 1%
most cited scientists

12.2%
Contributors from top 500 universities

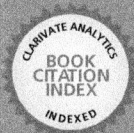

Interested in publishing with us?
Contact book.department@intechopen.com

Meet the editor

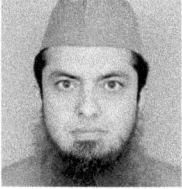

Dr. Rizwan Ahmad, a biochemist, currently serves as a University Professor in the College of Medicine at Imam Abdulrahman bin Faisal University in Dammam, Saudi Arabia. His academic journey began with a Master's and Doctorate from Aligarh Muslim University in Aligarh, India. During his Ph.D., he was awarded a prestigious scholarship from the Indian Council of Medical Research (ICMR) and the Council of Scientific Research (CSIR) in India. He also served as an Associate Professor at the National University of Oman and SBS University in Dehradun, India. Dr. Ahmad's research, which focuses on the role of free radicals in autoimmunity, has made significant contributions to the field. His findings are reflected in his numerous published research articles, chapters, and edited books.

Contents

Preface

Systemic lupus erythematosus (SLE) is the most prevalent form of lupus, affecting 7 out of 10 individuals diagnosed with the condition. This is what people typically refer to when they mention "lupus". The exact cause of SLE remains unknown to experts. However, many scientists believe that it develops due to a combination of internal and external factors.

SLE is a chronic autoimmune disease that decisively impacts multiple systems in the body and follows a relapsing and remitting course. Its prevalence is significantly higher in women of childbearing age, with a striking female-to-male ratio of approximately 9:1. Environmental and genetic factors unequivocally interact to trigger immune responses, leading to the excessive production of pathogenic autoantibodies by B cells and severe cytokine dysregulation. This ultimately causes significant tissue and organ damage. A defining characteristic of SLE is the presence of antibodies against nuclear and cytoplasmic antigens, underscoring its complexity and specialty.

The management and long-term complications of lupus have significantly improved over the past two decades; however, many critical questions about the disease remain unanswered. This underscores the urgent need for ongoing research. Effective management of lupus demands exceptional compliance and commitment from patients. Poor adherence to medication, inadequate monitoring, and failure to reassess disease activity typically result in poor outcomes, frequent relapses, and resistance cases. Patients must be thoroughly counseled about the disease's pathology, signs, and symptoms, the necessity of regular monitoring, and medication adherence. Additionally, preventive measures such as lifestyle changes, dietary modifications, and regular exercise must be emphasized to effectively control weight, manage lipid levels, and prevent cardiovascular complications.

Until now, all therapies for lupus have been generalized and non-specific, primarily involving broad immunosuppression. This approach makes it difficult to pinpoint the exact causes of the disease. Identifying these causes could lead to potential cures that do not carry the side effects associated with current treatments.

The book *Lupus – Diagnostics and Developments* provides a comprehensive overview of systemic lupus erythematosus (SLE) and explores various diagnostic methods. It also examines some of the latest techniques that may be essential for studying clinical and biological parameters. Furthermore, the book discusses placental malperfusion in mothers with SLE, a common complication, to offer insights into ongoing research in this area.

The task of editing this book would not have been completed without the invaluable support of Dr. Ghada F. Yousif and other colleagues at the College of Medicine. I also extend my special thanks to my family for their unwavering support throughout this journey. Additionally, I am grateful to Ms. Iva Horvat, the process manager at IntechOpen, for her guidance from start to finish. Above all, I thank Almighty for giving me the strength to complete this book project.

Dr. Rizwan Ahmad
College of Medicine,
Imam Abdulrahman Bin Faisal University,
Dammam, Saudi Arabia

Chapter 1

Introductory Chapter: Systemic Lupus Erythematosus – Basics and Developments

Mohammad Yusuf Hasan and Rizwan Ahmad

1. Introduction

Autoimmune diseases present an opportunity to understand the body's immune system better. In these conditions, the immune system mistakenly attacks its tissues, offering insights into the intricate workings of the immune system. This occurrence provides an avenue for further exploration into the adaptive immune system's recognition of self-antigens as foreign, potentially leading to advancements in treatment and management. Genetic predisposition and environmental factors offer promising areas for research and understanding the development of autoimmune diseases. Furthermore, investigating the triggers, including infections and ecological factors, holds the potential for identifying preventive measures and innovative treatment approaches. Systemic lupus erythematosus (SLE), a type of lupus characterized by inflammation, serves as a focal point for delving into the complexities of autoimmunity. In this chapter, we will delve into the basics of autoimmunity, explore the mechanisms behind lupus, and discuss recent updates in its understanding and management [1].

2. Understanding autoimmunity

The immune system is like a sophisticated puzzle of cells, tissues, and organs. Our bodies depend on it to shield us from harmful substances such as viruses, bacteria, and toxins. It achieves this by identifying and eliminating these invaders while protecting our cells and tissues.

Autoimmunity is a condition in which the immune system tragically loses its ability to distinguish between self and non-self-antigens, harming the body's tissues. While the exact cause of this disruption is not completely understood, it is thought to result from a combination of genetic predisposition, environmental factors, and immune system dysregulation [2].

3. Systemic lupus erythematosus

Systemic lupus erythematosus (SLE), commonly known as lupus, is an intricate autoimmune disease that can impact multiple organs and systems in the body [3].

IntechOpen

It is identified by periods of exacerbation and remission, with symptoms varying from mild to severe. The defining feature of SLE is the production of autoantibodies targeting various self-antigens, including DNA, RNA, and cell nuclear proteins. Autoantibodies form immune complexes that deposit in tissues, leading to inflammation and tissue damage [4].

Despite the complexity, ongoing efforts to comprehend SLE's pathogenesis and root causes are in progress. The biomarkers available for clinical use are currently limited, primarily encompassing anti-dsDNA antibodies, complement molecules, and white blood cell counts [5]. Distinguishing SLE from other conditions with similar presentations, such as rheumatoid arthritis (RA) and myositis, presents a challenge due to the array of symptoms. However, early detection and timely intervention can mitigate SLE relapses, reduce hospitalization rates, and minimize chronic organ damage [6]. Therefore, it is imperative to identify dependable biomarkers and unravel underlying molecular mechanisms to enhance SLE diagnosis and facilitate effective treatment.

The latest research breakthroughs have yielded crucial insights into the pathogenesis of SLE, paving the way for the creation of cutting-edge diagnostic and therapeutic approaches. Some recent updates include:

3.1 Genetic studies

Genome-wide association studies (GWAS) have uncovered numerous genetic variants associated with SLE susceptibility, shedding light on the genetic basis of the disease. SLE develops when individuals with genetic predisposition encounter specific environmental triggers, such as infectious agents, producing antinuclear antibodies (ANA). Following the emergence of ANA, there is a variable interval before immune material accumulates in tissue without concurrent inflammatory reactions [7].

SLE involves a complex interplay of multiple genes. Through a combination of genome-wide association studies (GWAS) and targeted gene investigations, over 40 robust genetic links to SLE have been identified. These genes regulate the expression of proteins crucial in various disease pathways, including apoptosis, clearance of apoptotic substances or immune complexes, innate and adaptive immunity functions, and the synthesis of cytokines, chemokines, and adhesion molecules [8].

3.2 Immunological mechanisms

Advances in the field of immunology have uncovered intricate pathways associated with the dysregulation of the immune system in SLE, shedding light on the roles of cytokines, B cells, and T cells. Extensive research has delved into the dysregulated immune response characteristic of SLE, encompassing both innate and adaptive immunity. Substantial progress has been made in elucidating the cellular and molecular underpinnings of SLE pathogenesis. B lymphocytes are instrumental in the adaptive immune response of SLE, contributing to the generation of autoantibodies, presentation of autoantigens, and activation of autoreactive T cells [9]. Additionally, T lymphocytes play a crucial role through co-stimulatory signals and cytokine secretion from specific T cell subsets. The involvement of innate immune responses in SLE pathogenesis, particularly the discovery of Toll-like receptors (TLRs) on plasmacytoid dendritic cells (pDCs) capable of being triggered by immune complexes, leading to IFN-α production and formation of neutrophil extracellular traps (NETs), has garnered attention [10]. These dysfunctions coexist and synergize, illustrating the interconnectedness of these factors and the locations of pertinent therapeutic targets. Understanding the immune pathophysiology of SLE has spurred the development of novel biologic agents aimed at selectively targeting aberrant immune processes, thereby mitigating the adverse effects associated with conventional broad-spectrum immunosuppressive therapies [11].

3.3 Biomarkers

Researchers have made significant progress in identifying biomarkers that have the potential to revolutionize the diagnosis, prognosis, and monitoring of SLE, paving the way for personalized management approaches. The complex and diverse nature of SLE has presented challenges in diagnosis, management, and research. However, ongoing investigations into various biomarker techniques, including DNA, messenger RNA, microRNA, antibody microarrays, flow cytometry, and proteomic markers, offer promising avenues for improvement. While current biomarker studies primarily focus on peripheral blood and urine samples, exploring other accessible tissues holds great potential. Although there is still a need for further research and rigorous multicenter validation studies, the growing pool of potential biomarkers for SLE is a positive step forward [12].

Identifying robust immunological markers is crucial for gaining deeper insights into disease progression in SLE patients, encompassing non-organ-specific and organ-specific biomarkers. It is essential to recognize that individual biomarkers may not possess the required sensitivity and specificity for SLE diagnosis, making the integration of multiple markers through mathematical models a promising approach for comprehensive SLE assessment. Moreover, leveraging advanced computational techniques to analyze extensive datasets will be instrumental in uncovering novel biomarkers for SLE [13].

3.4 Therapeutic developments

Investigating targeted therapies, such as biologics and small molecule inhibitors, provides promising results in controlling disease activity while minimizing side effects compared to traditional immunosuppressive agents. The updated recommendations from the European League Against Rheumatism (EULAR) for managing SLE emphasize hydroxychloroquine, glucocorticoids, immunosuppressive drugs, and biologics, offering a more comprehensive approach to treatment. Although the management of SLE has yet to make significant progress in replacing traditional therapies, recent guidelines from EULAR highlight the objective of achieving remission or low disease activity through treatment. The extension of the "treat-to-target" approach to SLE treatment strategies shows a promising shift in managing the condition. Regular updates from EULAR and the American College of Rheumatology (ACR) ensure that treatment strategies for SLE remain at the forefront of medical advancements [13, 14].

When considering pharmacotherapy using conventional disease-modifying drugs (csDMARDs), it is advisable to utilize hydroxychloroquine (HCQ) for all patients at a dosage not exceeding 5 mg/kg of body weight to minimize the risk of retinal complications. HCQ has a well-established long-term safety profile and has been proven to reduce disease flares and cardiovascular events [15–17]. Its affordability makes it suitable even in low-income regions, highlighting its continued importance in SLE treatment alongside innovative medications. For long-term management, it is recommended to gradually reduce glucocorticoid doses to less than 7.5 mg/day prednisone equivalent and, if feasible, discontinue them due to the adverse effects associated with long-term or high-dose use. These effects may include osteoporosis, exacerbation of diabetes and hypertension, and increased susceptibility to infections [18].

In some instances, steroid-sparing agents, such as azathioprine, methotrexate, mycophenolate mofetil, and cyclophosphamide (CYC), have the potential to allow for the discontinuation of steroids. However, their usage is constrained by side effects and toxicity. Mycophenolate, which has shown greater efficacy than azathioprine, is not recommended during pregnancy due to its potential to cause congenital disabilities. Despite its effectiveness in treating severe organ-related issues, such as central nervous system involvement and lupus nephritis (LN), CYC is linked to significant side effects, including an increased risk of cancer. Therefore, there is an apparent demand for new therapies for patients who do not respond well to conventional immunosuppressants or for those who require safer treatment options during pregnancy [19–21].

While reducing steroid usage is essential, steroids remain a crucial part of the treatment. Additionally, traditional immunosuppressive therapies continue to be essential. Therefore, considering innovative or biological drugs is advised only when conventional treatment fails to adequately manage the disease [21].

4. Conclusion

Systemic lupus erythematosus is a multifaceted autoimmune condition with a wide range of clinical symptoms, significantly affecting the quality of life for those it afflicts. Despite significant strides in comprehending its underlying mechanisms and creating innovative treatment approaches, further investigation is necessary to understand its intricacies completely. With continuous progress in the field, there is optimism for enhanced outcomes and improved management of SLE in the times ahead.

Acknowledgements

The author used Generative AI from the Grammarly website for the language polishing of the manuscript.

Author details

Mohammad Yusuf Hasan[1] and Rizwan Ahmad[2*]

1 Centre for Drug and Herbal Development, Faculty of Pharmacy, Universiti Kebangsaan Malaysia, Kuala Lumpur, Malaysia

2 College of Medicine, Imam Abdulrahman Bin Faisal University, Dammam, Saudi Arabia

*Address all correspondence to: ahmadriz.biochem@gmail.com

IntechOpen

References

[1] Ballotti S, Chiarelli F, de Martino M. Autoimmunity: Basic mechanisms and implications in endocrine diseases: Part I. Hormone Research. 2006;**66**(3):132-141

[2] Land WG. Basic trajectories in autoimmunity. In: Damage-Associated Molecular Patterns in Human Diseases: Volume 3: Antigen-Related Disorders. Cham: Springer International Publishing; 2023. pp. 383-456

[3] Tsokos GC. Systemic lupus erythematosus. The New England Journal of Medicine. 2011;**365**(22):2110-2121

[4] Pons-Estel GJ et al. Understanding the epidemiology and progression of systemic lupus erythematosus. Seminars in Arthritis and Rheumatism. 2010;**39**(4):257-268

[5] Piga M, Arnaud L. The main challenges in systemic lupus erythematosus: Where do we stand? Journal of Clinical Medicine. 2021;**10**(2):243

[6] Mak A, Isenberg DA, Lau C-S. Global trends, potential mechanisms and early detection of organ damage in SLE. Nature Reviews Rheumatology. 2013;**9**(5):301-310

[7] Delgado-Vega A et al. Recent findings on genetics of systemic autoimmune diseases. Current Opinion in Immunology. 2010;**22**(6):698-705

[8] Rhodes B, Vyse TJ. The genetics of SLE: An update in the light of genome-wide association studies. Rheumatology (Oxford). 2008;**47**(11):1603-1611

[9] Fillatreau S et al. B cells regulate autoimmunity by provision of IL-10. Nature Immunology. 2002;**3**(10):944-950

[10] Katsuyama T, Tsokos GC, Moulton VR. Aberrant T cell signaling and subsets in systemic lupus erythematosus. Frontiers in Immunology. 2018;**9**:1088

[11] Pan L et al. Immunological pathogenesis and treatment of systemic lupus erythematosus. World Journal of Pediatrics. 2020;**16**(1):19-30

[12] Yu H, Nagafuchi Y, Fujio K. Clinical and immunological biomarkers for systemic lupus erythematosus. Biomolecules. 2021;**11**(7):928

[13] van Vollenhoven R et al. A framework for remission in SLE: Consensus findings from a large international task force on definitions of remission in SLE (DORIS). Annals of the Rheumatic Diseases. 2017;**76**(3):554-561

[14] Franklyn K et al. Definition and initial validation of a lupus low disease activity state (LLDAS). Annals of the Rheumatic Diseases. 2016;**75**(9):1615-1621

[15] Almeida-Brasil CC et al. Flares after hydroxychloroquine reduction or discontinuation: Results from the systemic lupus international collaborating clinics (SLICC) inception cohort. Annals of the Rheumatic Diseases. 2022;**81**(3):370-378

[16] Shinjo SK et al. Antimalarial treatment may have a time-dependent effect on lupus survival: Data from a multinational Latin American inception cohort. Arthritis & Rheumatism. 2010;**62**(3):855-862

[17] Ruiz-Irastorza G et al. Clinical efficacy and side effects of antimalarials in systemic lupus erythematosus:

A systematic review. Annals of the
Rheumatic Diseases. 2010;**69**(1):20-28

[18] Ugarte-Gil MF et al. Impact of
glucocorticoids on the incidence of
lupus-related major organ damage: A
systematic literature review and meta-
regression analysis of longitudinal
observational studies. Lupus Science &
Medicine. 2021;**8**(1):e000590

[19] Anderka MT et al. Reviewing the
evidence for mycophenolate mofetil
as a new teratogen: Case report and
review of the literature. American
Journal of Medical Genetics. Part A.
2009;**149a**(6):1241-1248

[20] Houssiau FA et al.
Immunosuppressive therapy in lupus
nephritis: The euro-lupus nephritis
trial, a randomized trial of low-
dose versus high-dose intravenous
cyclophosphamide. Arthritis and
Rheumatism. 2002;**46**(8):2121-2131

[21] Dörner T, Furie R. Novel paradigms
in systemic lupus erythematosus. Lancet.
2019;**393**(10188):2344-2358

Chapter 2

Immunological Biomarkers as an Effective Means for Diagnosing Systemic Lupus Erythematosus (SLE)

Rizwan Ahmad

Abstract

Systemic lupus erythematosus (SLE) is an autoimmune disease that relentlessly attacks the body's tissues, leading to widespread inflammation and consequential tissue damage in various organs, including the joints, skin, brain, lungs, kidneys, and blood vessels. While there is no known cure for this disease, it can be managed effectively through medical interventions and lifestyle modifications. It is imperative to note that SLE can significantly impact an individual's quality of life, both in the short and long term. Diagnosing and assessing pathophysiological processes in SLE using clinical and physiological assessments alone is often inadequate. Immunological biomarkers show promise in enhancing SLE diagnosis, assessment, and management. Early detection of SLE is crucial for effective treatment. Thus, biomarkers, particularly immunological biomarkers, have emerged as a potential solution to improve the diagnosis and assessment of SLE's pathophysiological processes. The ultimate aim is to improve disease control. This chapter comprehensively reviews immunological biomarkers for SLE diagnosis and pathophysiological aspects.

Keywords: systemic lupus erythematosus, biomarkers, antinuclear antibodies, anti-double-stranded DNA antibodies, pathophysiology

1. Introduction

The clinical presentations of systemic lupus erythematosus (SLE) exhibit significant diversity, with individuals showcasing varying symptoms over time. This diversity poses a considerable challenge in diagnosing and monitoring disease activity [1]. Presently, the primary immunological markers for diagnosing SLE include anti-double-stranded DNA (anti-dsDNA) antibodies, antinuclear antibodies, and anti-Smith (anti-SM) antibodies [2]. However, their sensitivity and specificity need to be improved, leaving room for enhanced diagnostic accuracy. Therefore, it is crucial to investigate the characteristic genes linked to the development and advancement of SLE [3].

Biomarkers, also known as biological markers, are not just tools for diagnosis, but they play a crucial role in various aspects of disease management. They are measurable

IntechOpen

characteristics that objectively evaluate and indicate normal biological processes, pathogenic processes, or responses to a therapeutic intervention. They are of different types, including prognostic, diagnostic, predictive, pharmacodynamic, and surrogate biomarkers. Prognostic biomarkers help identify individuals at risk of developing a disease or those likely to experience a flare. Diagnostic biomarkers confirm the presence or subtype of a disease. Predictive biomarkers use baseline characteristics to predict therapeutic responses. Pharmacodynamic biomarkers help determine optimal therapeutic doses. Finally, surrogate biomarkers replace a clinical endpoint [4–6].

In recent years, technologies such as next-generation sequencing and mass spectrometry have shown promising results in identifying new biomarkers for assessing disease activity and diagnosing SLE. Various prediction methods for SLE have also emerged with the advancement of bioinformatics. Early diagnosis of SLE is crucial for effective treatment. Therefore, immunological biomarkers have become a promising tool for early SLE diagnosis and assessment of its pathophysiological processes, to improve disease control.

2. Antinuclear antibodies (ANA)

ANA, autoantibodies directed against nuclear antigens, including double-stranded DNA (dsDNA), histones, and nucleosomes, are highly sensitive but less specific markers for SLE. Their presence in other autoimmune diseases and infections can lead to false positives. However, ANA testing remains a crucial step in the initial evaluation of suspected SLE cases, underscoring its importance in the diagnostic process [7].

The detection of antinuclear antibodies (ANA) through indirect immunofluorescence (IIF) on HEp-2 cells has long been recognized as a crucial immunological marker in serum for identifying patients with systemic lupus erythematosus (SLE) and for evaluating their suitability for SLE diagnosis [8–10]. The ANA test is incorporated into the criteria of ACR-1997, SLICC-2012, and EULAR/ACR-2019 [11, 12]. According to the EULAR/ACR-2019 criteria, a minimum IIF-ANA titer of 1:80 is required for diagnosing SLE [12]. If ANA is positive, additional testing for antigen-specific ANAs like dsDNA, SSA (Ro60), Sjögren's syndrome antigen B, Sm, and ribonuclear protein is recommended. While ANA's presence is not exclusive to SLE, it strongly suggests it and serves various purposes such as screening, classification, diagnosis, prognosis, and staging [8, 13]. ANA tests exhibit high sensitivity (90 to 95%) in SLE patients but relatively low specificity, occurring in 5–20% of healthy individuals, particularly in the elderly [14]. The sensitivity of ANA tests may aid in early SLE detection [15]. However, a negative ANA test does not rule out SLE, with studies indicating ANA negativity in a small percentage of SLE patients, even up to 30% in clinical trials for new therapies [13, 16]. Discrepancies in ANA results in SLE may stem from variations in IIF-ANA assays, differences in antigen properties, effects of HEp-2 cells on nuclear antigens, laboratory protocols, or interpretation thresholds [9, 17]. Thus, establishing a standardized ANA test with consistent specificity, detection methods, and laboratory procedures is imperative for the future.

3. Anti-dsDNA antibodies

Anti-dsDNA antibodies are particularly associated with SLE and disease activity, especially lupus nephritis. Detecting these antibodies using techniques such as enzyme-linked immunosorbent assay (ELISA) or immunofluorescence assays can assist in diagnosing and monitoring SLE.

The presence of these antibodies is a critical diagnostic feature and is included in the ACR, SLICC, and the 2019 EULAR/ACR classification criteria for SLE [18, 19]. They can be found in up to 70% of SLE patients and have a 96% specificity for SLE. These antibodies typically appear early in the development of SLE and may even precede its official diagnosis, especially in patients with lupus nephritis (LN). However, their diagnostic sensitivity ranges from 52 to 70% due to their transient nature, variability in laboratory assays used for detection, and the specific isotypes targeted [20]. The main methods for detecting anti-dsDNA antibodies are enzyme-linked immunosorbent assay (ELISA) and immunofluorescence using Crithidia luciliae as a substrate. The Farr radioimmunoassay (RIA) technique has become less common in laboratories due to its use of radiolabeled reagents [20].

4. Complement proteins

Complement proteins, such as C3 and C4, are crucial in the immune response and are often depleted in patients with active SLE due to complement activation and consumption. Low levels of C3 and C4 complement proteins are linked to disease activity and can aid in diagnosing SLE when combined with other serological tests.

Immune complexes can activate complement [21]. Serum levels of C3 and C4 are commonly used to assess the presence of biologically active immune complexes [22] and to monitor disease activity. Reduced serum levels of C3 or C4 are considered immunological markers in the SLICC-2012 classification criteria for SLE. According to the immunological criteria, decreased levels of both C3 and C4 carry more weight than having low levels of either C3 or C4 alone in the EULAR/ACR-2019 classification criteria for SLE [23]. Patients with low levels of both C3 and C4 are more likely to be diagnosed with SLE than those with low levels of C3 or C4 alone. Patients with either low C3 or low C4 along with a positive ANA test have a specificity of 94.3% for an SLE diagnosis, whereas patients with concurrently low C3 and C4 levels alongside a positive ANA have a specificity of 97.6% for an SLE diagnosis [24]. Furthermore, decreased levels of C3 and C4 can precede a clinically evident flare and are positively correlated with SLE disease activity [25], especially in cases of SLE complicated by renal or hematologic flares [26]. However, due to the limited specificity of C3 and C4 in SLE diagnosis, their reliability as biomarkers can be limited when used alone, especially in certain patients [27].

5. B cell and T cell biomarkers

The activation and differentiation of abnormal B and T cells are crucial to SLE development. Biomarkers such as CD19 + CD20+ B cells, CD4+ T cells, and regulatory T cells (Tregs) have been linked to SLE pathogenesis and may be potential targets for treatment. In the pathogenesis of SLE, similar to other autoimmune conditions, the breakdown of tolerance in both T and B cells is fundamental. Recent studies on the immunopathogenesis of SLE suggest that specific individuals have a genetic predisposition to losing tolerance to self-antigens, leading to abnormal T cells and excessive production of autoantibodies. This ultimately results in tissue and organ damage caused by autoreactive B lymphocytes [28, 29]. T cells from SLE patients show various abnormalities in terms of their characteristics and numbers, contributing to the development of SLE and providing potentially valuable biomarkers [30].

Key T cell subsets implicated in SLE include T-helper cell type 1 (Th1), T-helper cell type 2 (Th2), Th17 cells, follicular T cells (Tfh), and T-regulatory (Treg) cells. T cells from individuals with SLE exhibit increased resistance to apoptosis induction by thymic stromal cells [31]. The T-cell receptor (TCR) complex on T lymphocyte surfaces consists of the TCR, CD3, and the zeta chain. Functionally, T cells are categorized into T helper cells (CD4+) and cytotoxic T lymphocytes (CD8+). T lymphocyte activation is characterized by the expression of various antigens, including HLA-DR. The activation and differentiation of abnormal B and T cells are crucial to SLE development. Biomarkers such as CD19 + CD20+ B cells, CD4+ T cells, and regulatory T cells (Tregs) have been linked to SLE pathogenesis and may be potential targets for treatment [32].

6. Erythrocyte sedimentation rate (ESR) and C-reactive protein (CRP)

While oligoclonal and monoclonal gammopathies can occur in SLE patients, they are not the norm or directly attributed to SLE. On the other hand, polyclonal hyper-gammaglobulinemia is common in SLE, which aligns with the nature of an autoan-tibody-mediated disease [33]. Hypergammaglobulinemia reflects heightened B and plasma cell activity, indicating autoimmunity rather than inflammation. Although IL-6 stimulates B cells, most pro-inflammatory cytokines tend to limit rather than enhance polyclonal antibody production. Therefore, we must look at other abundant proteins to indicate inflammatory disease. Fibrinogen, typically elevated during inflammation as part of the acute phase response, shows only mild increases in SLE compared to other inflammatory disorders [34].

Furthermore, unlike in different conditions, fibrinogen levels do not seem to correlate with IL-6 in lupus inflammation [35]. Conversely, low fibrinogen levels may occasionally occur due to intravascular activation of the coagulation cascade but would not significantly raise the ESR. Therefore, fibrinogen likely does not substantially contribute to the increased ESR in active SLE.

The level of plasma albumin has an opposite effect on the erythrocyte sedimentation rate (ESR) compared to fibrinogen. Adequate levels of albumin tend to lower the ESR, while reduced albumin production raises it. In SLE patients, plasma albumin levels are notably reduced compared to healthy individuals, especially in those with active SLE compared to inactive disease. Inflammation can directly impede albumin production in the liver as part of the acute phase response. Additionally, reduced appetite, influenced by elevated TNF levels, may play a significant role. Both mechanisms may be pertinent in active SLE. However, the primary factor in reducing serum albumin is likely renal albumin loss through damaged glomeruli, as suggested by the stronger association in patients with lupus nephritis [22]. The impact of diminished albumin on the ESR thus represents an initial inflammatory component.

CRP is the standard indicator of inflammation, but in SLE patients, it tends to function more as an indicator of severe infections. CRP levels are directly influenced by IL-6 [36], with increased IL-6 levels observed in active SLE [37, 38]. Consequently, CRP levels often deviate from the normal range in active SLE [39]. Elevated CRP levels are typically observed in patients experiencing active serositis arthritis or myositis. In most other scenarios, CRP levels remain below 60 mg/L or 6 mg/dL during active SLE [40]. Levels exceeding this threshold are more indicative of severe infections. CRP values reaching 150 mg/L or 15 mg/dL strongly suggest the presence of infections, while levels of 20 mg/L (2 mg/dL) CRP or lower indicate a lower likelihood of infection [41]. This distinction holds clinical significance as severe infections significantly contribute to mortality among SLE patients [42–44].

7. Cytokines and chemokines

When considering SLE activity, it is essential to consider various cytokines beyond the standard markers. These encompass type I interferons, particularly IFNα and IL-6, IL-10, IL-15, IL-18, BAFF/BLyS, and TNF [45–47]. IFNα is primarily produced by plasmacytoid dendritic cells (pDC) [48], while monocytes and macrophages largely synthesize the other mentioned cytokines. Notably, T cell cytokines like IFNγ, which act more locally, are typically not measurable in significant quantities. Among the elevated cytokines in SLE, IL-10, IL-15, and BAFF/BLyS mainly serve an immunoregulatory rather than inflammatory function [48].

Chemokines in serum or plasma, much like cytokines, can be conveniently measured using ELISA technology. While chemokines are generally produced in response to cytokines and serve as more indirect markers of the inflammatory process, there is evidence linking them to disease activity. CCL2/MCP-1, CXCCL10/IP-10, and CCL19 are recognized as interferon-inducible genes, leading to the development of a composite score to estimate interferon activity associated with SLE disease activity, similar to the interferon signature mentioned earlier. Previous studies have found elevated levels of CCL2 and CXCL10 in active SLE, suggesting that these chemokines may provide insight into the influence of interferons in SLE. Additionally, CCL-11, CXCL13, and CXCL16 have been associated with disease activity, while serum IL-8, CCL17, CXCL16, and CX3CL1 have been linked to active lupus nephritis [48].

8. Clinical significance of immunological biomarkers

8.1 Early diagnosis and disease monitoring

Immunological biomarkers are essential for early SLE diagnosis, enabling prompt treatment initiation and improved disease management. Monitoring changes in biomarker levels over time can help evaluate disease activity, predict flares, and inform treatment decisions [49].

8.2 Predicting disease manifestations

Specific immunological biomarkers, such as anti-dsDNA antibodies and complement proteins, are linked to particular disease manifestations in SLE, such as lupus nephritis and neuropsychiatric symptoms. Understanding these connections can assist clinicians in predicting disease outcomes and implementing suitable interventions [49].

8.3 Personalized medicine

Identifying specific immunological biomarker profiles in individual patients can facilitate personalized treatment strategies in SLE. Customizing treatment based on biomarker profiles may enhance treatment response rates, reduce adverse effects, and optimize long-term outcomes [50].

8.4 Prognostic indicators

Immunological biomarkers aid in diagnosis and disease monitoring and serve as prognostic indicators for SLE outcomes. Elevated levels of specific biomarkers, such as anti-dsDNA antibodies and pro-inflammatory cytokines, have increased disease severity, organ damage, and mortality [50].

9. Challenges and future directions

The field of immunological biomarkers has seen significant advancements, yet there are still challenges in their practical use for SLE diagnosis and management. These challenges present opportunities for improvement, including the standardization of assays, addressing variations in biomarker expression, and conducting further validation studies to ensure reliability and reproducibility.

Moving forward, research efforts can focus on identifying and developing novel biomarkers with enhanced sensitivity and specificity for SLE. Understanding the mechanisms underlying biomarker dysregulation and leveraging this knowledge to develop targeted therapies based on biomarker profiles is crucial. Additionally, integrating multi-omics approaches, such as genomics, transcriptomics, and proteomics, holds promise in providing a more comprehensive understanding of SLE and uncovering new biomarkers and therapeutic targets.

10. Conclusion

Immunological biomarkers have revolutionized Systemic Lupus Erythematosus (SLE) diagnosis and management. These biomarkers provide crucial information about the disease's underlying causes and help predict the progression and severity of the condition. Furthermore, they are pivotal in tailoring treatment strategies to suit individual patients, leading to more personalized and effective care. By harnessing the latest immunology and molecular biology breakthroughs, we are continually advancing our knowledge of SLE and developing cutting-edge biomarkers and targeted therapies to improve patient outcomes.

Acknowledgements

The author used Generative AI from the Grammarly website for the language polishing of the manuscript.

Author details

Rizwan Ahmad
College of Medicine, Imam Abdulrahman Bin Faisal University, Dammam,
Saudi Arabia

*Address all correspondence to: ahmadriz.biochem@gmail.com

IntechOpen

References

[1] Basta F et al. Systemic lupus erythematosus (SLE) therapy: The old and the new. Rheumatology and Therapy. 2020;**7**(3):433-446

[2] Lee J-M et al. Novel immunoprofiling method for diagnosing SLE and evaluating therapeutic response. Lupus Science & Medicine. 2022;**9**(1):e000693

[3] Arriens C, Wren JD, Munroe ME, Mohan C. Systemic lupus erythematosus biomarkers: The challenging quest. Rheumatology (Oxford, England). 2017;**56**(Suppl. 1):i32

[4] Ahmad R, Ahsan H. Peroxynitrite modified antigen-immunological marker in systemic lupus erythematosus. In: Chapter in Recent Developments in Biotechnology, Biotechnology Series. Vol. 5. Houston, USA: Studium Press; 2014

[5] Ahmad R, Sah AK, Ahsan H. Peroxynitrite modified photoadducts as possible pathophysiological biomarkers: A short review. Journal of Molecular Biomarkers & Diagnosis. 2015;**6**:263

[6] He J et al. Serum proteome and metabolome uncover novel biomarkers for the assessment of disease activity and diagnosing of systemic lupus erythematosus. Clinical Immunology. 2023;**251**:109330

[7] Wu FL et al. Identification of serum biomarkers for systemic lupus erythematosus using a library of phage displayed random peptides and deep sequencing. Molecular & Cellular Proteomics. 2019;**18**(9):1851-1863

[8] Damoiseaux J et al. Clinical relevance of HEp-2 indirect immunofluorescent patterns: The international consensus on ANA patterns (ICAP) perspective. Annals of the Rheumatic Diseases. 2019;**78**(7):879-889

[9] Olsen NJ, Karp DR. Autoantibodies and SLE—The threshold for disease. Nature Reviews Rheumatology. 2014;**10**(3):181-186

[10] Meroni PL, Schur PH. ANA screening: An old test with new recommendations. Annals of the Rheumatic Diseases. 2010;**69**(8):1420-1422

[11] Tan EM et al. The 1982 revised criteria for the classification of systemic lupus erythematosus. Arthritis & Rheumatism: Official Journal of the American College of Rheumatology. 1982;**25**(11):1271-1277

[12] Aringer M et al. 2019 European league against rheumatism/American College of Rheumatology classification criteria for systemic lupus erythematosus. Arthritis and Rheumatology. 2019;**71**(9):1400-1412

[13] Pisetsky DS. Antinuclear antibody testing—Misunderstood or misbegotten? Nature Reviews Rheumatology. 2017;**13**(8):495-502

[14] Emlen W, O'Neill L. Clinical significance of antinuclear antibodies. Comparison of detection with immunofluorescence and enzyme-linked immunosorbent assays. Arthritis & Rheumatism: Official Journal of the American College of Rheumatology. 1997;**40**(9):1612-1618

[15] Sjöwall C et al. Abnormal antinuclear antibody titers are less common than generally assumed in established cases of systemic lupus erythematosus. The Journal of Rheumatology. 2008;**35**(10):1994-2000

[16] Choi MY et al. Antinuclear antibody–negative systemic lupus erythematosus in an international inception cohort. Arthritis Care & Research. 2019;**71**(7):893-902

[17] Pisetsky DS, Lipsky PE. New insights into the role of antinuclear antibodies in systemic lupus erythematosus. Nature Reviews Rheumatology. 2020;**16**(10):565-579

[18] Amezcua-Guerra LM et al. Performance of the 2012 systemic lupus international collaborating clinics and the 1997 American College of Rheumatology classification criteria for systemic lupus erythematosus in a real-life scenario. Arthritis Care & Research (Hoboken). 2015;**67**(3):437-441

[19] Reveille JD. Predictive value of autoantibodies for activity of systemic lupus erythematosus. Lupus. 2004;**13**(5):290-297

[20] Petri M et al. Derivation and validation of the systemic lupus international collaborating clinics classification criteria for systemic lupus erythematosus. Arthritis and Rheumatism. 2012;**64**(8):2677-2686

[21] Leffler J, Bengtsson AA, Blom AM. The complement system in systemic lupus erythematosus: An update. Annals of the Rheumatic Diseases. 2014;**73**(9):1601-1606

[22] Trouw LA, Pickering MC, Blom AM. The complement system as a potential therapeutic target in rheumatic disease. Nature Reviews Rheumatology. 2017;**13**(9):538-547

[23] Sacre K et al. New 2019 SLE EULAR/ACR classification criteria are valid for identifying patients with SLE among patients admitted for pericardial effusion. Annals of the Rheumatic Diseases. 2021;**80**(12):e190-e190

[24] Li H et al. Diagnostic value of serum complement C3 and C4 levels in Chinese patients with systemic lupus erythematosus. Clinical Rheumatology. 2015;**34**:471-477

[25] Petri MA et al. Baseline predictors of systemic lupus erythematosus flares: Data from the combined placebo groups in the phase III belimumab trials. Arthritis & Rheumatism. 2013;**65**(8):2143-2153

[26] Ho A et al. A decrease in complement is associated with increased renal and hematologic activity in patients with systemic lupus erythematosus. Arthritis & Rheumatism. 2001;**44**(10):2350-2357

[27] Larosa M et al. Advances in the diagnosis and classification of systemic lupus erythematosus. Expert Review of Clinical Immunology. 2016;**12**(12):1309-1320

[28] Sestak AL et al. The genetics of systemic lupus erythematosus and implications for targeted therapy. Annals of the Rheumatic Diseases. 2011;**70**(Suppl. 1):i37-i43

[29] Deng Y, Tsao BP. Advances in lupus genetics and epigenetics. Current Opinion in Rheumatology. 2014;**26**(5):482-492

[30] Hoffman RW. T cells in the pathogenesis of systemic lupus erythematosus. Clinical Immunology. 2004;**113**(1):4-13

[31] Yeoh S-A, Dias SS, Isenberg DA. Advances in systemic lupus erythematosus. Medicine. 2018;**46**(2):84-92

[32] Abbas AK, Lichtman AH, Pillai S. Cellular and Molecular Immunology. Brasil: Elsevier; 2007

[33] Cuadrado MJ et al. Immunoglobulin abnormalities are frequent in patients with lupus nephritis. BMC Rheumatology. 2019;3:30

[34] Ames PR et al. Fibrinogen in systemic lupus erythematosus: More than an acute phase reactant? The Journal of Rheumatology. 2000;27(5):1190-1195

[35] Gabay C et al. Absence of correlation between interleukin 6 and C-reactive protein blood levels in systemic lupus erythematosus compared with rheumatoid arthritis. The Journal of Rheumatology. 1993;20(5):815-821

[36] Szalai AJ et al. Testosterone and IL-6 requirements for human C-reactive protein gene expression in transgenic mice. Journal of Immunology. 1998;160(11):5294-5299

[37] Studnicka-Benke A et al. Tumour necrosis factor alpha and its soluble receptors parallel clinical disease and autoimmune activity in systemic lupus erythematosus. British Journal of Rheumatology. 1996;35(11):1067-1074

[38] Gröndal G et al. Cytokine production, serum levels and disease activity in systemic lupus erythematosus. Clinical and Experimental Rheumatology. 2000;18(5):565-570

[39] Becker GJ et al. Value of serum C-reactive protein measurement in the investigation of fever in systemic lupus erythematosus. Annals of the Rheumatic Diseases. 1980;39(1):50-52

[40] Ball EM et al. Plasma IL-6 levels correlate with clinical and ultrasound measures of arthritis in patients with systemic lupus erythematosus. Lupus. 2014;23(1):46-56

[41] Littlejohn E et al. The ratio of erythrocyte sedimentation rate to C-reactive protein is useful in distinguishing infection from flare in systemic lupus erythematosus patients presenting with fever. Lupus. 2018;27(7):1123-1129

[42] Anver H, Dubey S, Fox J. P51 trends in mortality in systemic lupus erythematosus: An analysis of SLE inpatient mortality at university hospital Coventry and warwickshire NHS trust from 2007-2016. Lupus Science & Medicine. 2020;7(Suppl. 1):A53-A53

[43] Tselios K et al. All-cause, cause-specific and age-specific standardised mortality ratios of patients with systemic lupus erythematosus in Ontario, Canada over 43 years (1971-2013). Annals of the Rheumatic Diseases. 2019;78(6):802-806

[44] Wu X-Y et al. Causes of death in hospitalized patients with systemic lupus erythematosus: A 10-year multicenter nationwide Chinese cohort. Clinical Rheumatology. 2019;38(1):107-115

[45] Idborg H et al. TNF-α and plasma albumin as biomarkers of disease activity in systemic lupus erythematosus. Lupus Science & Medicine. 2018;5(1):e000260

[46] Ytterberg SR, Schnitzer TJ. Serum interferon levels in patients with systemic lupus erythematosus. Arthritis & Rheumatism. 1982;25(4):401-406

[47] Petri M et al. Association of plasma B lymphocyte stimulator levels and disease activity in systemic lupus erythematosus. Arthritis and Rheumatism. 2008;58(8):2453-2459

[48] Banchereau J, Pascual V. Type I interferon in systemic lupus erythematosus and other autoimmune diseases. Immunity. 2006;25(3): 383-392

[49] Dörner T, Furie R. Novel paradigms
in systemic lupus erythematosus. Lancet.
2019;**393**(10188):2344-2358

[50] Akhil A et al. Systemic lupus
erythematosus: Latest insight into
etiopathogenesis. Rheumatology
International. 2023;**43**(8):1381-1393

Diagnosis and Management of GYn/Ob Manifestation of Systemic Lupus Erythematosus

Ismini Anagnostaki, Konstantinos Zacharis, Konstantia Loga and Ioannis Gkougkourelas

Abstract

Systemic lupus erythematosus (SLE), being an autoimmune disease with multisystem manifestations, poses significant challenges for women of reproductive age since infertility and increased risk of fetus loss reduce reproductive capacity. Furthermore, SLE seems to be associated with higher cancer probabilities of vulvar and vaginal cancers, as well as non-Hodgkin lymphoma (NHL) and lung cancer. Conversely, evidence suggests that ovarian and uterine cancers may exhibit a protective association with SLE. Through a review of current literature, we aim to elucidate the gynecological and obstetric manifestations and risks of SLE while proposing preventive and therapeutic strategies for this vulnerable patient population. Regarding cancer prevention, it is imperative to encourage SLE patients to undergo regular cancer screenings, consider human papilloma virus (HPV) vaccination, and adopt lifestyle modifications to mitigate known cancer risk factors such as smoking and obesity. During pregnancy, successful management entails meticulous planning and tailored medication strategies to minimize risks for both mother and fetus and mitigate the heightened risk of disease flare-ups typically associated with pregnancy. This comprehensive approach seeks to lessen the impact of cancer on SLE patients and enhance overall health outcomes. In general, we investigate the impact of SLE on the reproductive health of patients and the significant risk of malignant diseases later in woman's life.

Keywords: systemic lupus, antiphospholipid syndrome, gynecological cancers, infertility, obstetrics complications of SLE

1. Introduction

Systemic lupus erythematosus (SLE) is a multisystem autoimmune disease that most commonly affects young women of reproductive age. Even though SLE does not directly affect fertility, the prescribed medications may induce ovarian failure or exhibit teratogenic effects. In the past, women diagnosed with SLE were counseled against pregnancy due to concerns about potential complications for both the mother and the fetus. As time and therefore science progress, successful disease management offers the possibility of more favorable perinatal outcomes. Nevertheless, the young woman with SLE who wishes to become a mother faces several potential complications impacting both herself and the fetus. A severe flare-up of the disease can pose a potential risk to the mother's life, compounded by the fact that the administered drugs carry teratogenic and embryotoxic properties. Effective management involves early planning and ongoing vigilance in handling potential complications, as well as the careful administration and assessment of medications throughout the various stages of pregnancy. Additionally, some cases subsume additional risks such as renal failure and possible coexistence of antiphospholipid (aPL), anti-Ro, or anti-La antibodies. Furthermore, SLE and its treatment, notably, heighten the risk of gynecological malignancies, establishing the condition as a lifelong concern for women upon receiving the diagnosis.

2. SLE and fertility

While there is a consensus that patients with SLE generally exhibit fertility capacity similar to that of the general population, the onset of SLE diagnosis often correlates with a reduction in pregnancy rates. This decline in birth rate varies across different ethnic groups, with patients of Caucasian descent tending to have fewer offspring compared to similarly aged women. Infertility reported in SLE patients may arise from autoimmune mechanisms associated directly with the disease or as a side effect of treatment. Primary ovarian failure (POF) is a commonly encountered manifestation in patients with lupus, usually presenting as amenorrhea. Amenorrhea episodes have been associated with the presence of anti-corpus luteum antibodies and elevated follicular stimulating hormone (FSH) levels, suggesting an autoimmune, SLE-related dysfunction [1]. Menstrual disturbances are more likely to present in patients with high disease activity, as demonstrated by the systemic lupus erythematosus disease activity index score (SLEDAI5 8), than in those with lower disease activity levels. Interestingly, in this group of patients, there was no evidence of an association with hormonal disturbances, such as in the hypothalamic-pituitary axis, that could explain such a menstrual disturbance. Similarly, female patients with juvenile SLE have been reported to suffer from amenorrhea during periods of high disease activity. These patients have normal or even low FSH levels, in contrast to those with POF in whom FSH levels are elevated, raising the possibility that the cause of the menstrual disorder is due to the effects of the disease on the reproductive organs rather than a disorder of hypothalamic-pituitary axis Hashimoto's thyroiditis can be associated with SLE and can also cause menstrual disturbances, albeit through endocrine disruption [1].

Endometriosis leads to infertility through the development of adhesions that obstruct the fallopian tubes or impair follicular development, even in non-SLE patients. Several reports have identified immunological abnormalities in infertile patients with endometriosis, including both cell-mediated and humoral autoimmunity, indicating a potential association between autoantibodies and cell-mediated immune dysfunction in lupus-related infertility [2]. However, current data supporting the correlation between SLE and endometriosis remains controversial.

Given that some infections may contribute to infertility in the general population and the fact that SLE and/or immunosuppressive therapy may increase susceptibility to infections in exposed individuals, it is plausible that patients with SLE may exhibit an elevated risk of infertility due to infection [3]. Emerging evidence indicates the vulnerability of young women with SLE, particularly those with a higher SLEDAI DAS, to sexually transmitted infections. Although cytomegalovirus (CMV) and Epstein-Barr virus (EBV) infections are more common in lupus patients and have been implicated in infertility, specific evidence linking these infections to infertility in lupus patients is currently lacking. Another major cause of infertility affecting the general population, *Chlamydia trachomatis*, is still being researched regarding its impact on fertility in SLE patients. It is imperative to identify patients with SLE who may be prone to sexually transmitted infections and refer them for appropriate testing and treatment.

Cyclophosphamide (CYC) induced POF is associated with sustained high FSH levels. CYC, a well-known gonadotoxic agent, may lead to POF by depleting healthy oocytes. Its toxicity is associated with two independent risk factors: the cumulative dose of CYC and the age at which the drug is administered. Boumpas et al. showed that increasing age and dose of CYC are significant risk factors for POF, with a number of other studies supporting the same hypothesis [4–9]. Patients who receive cyclophosphamide at a younger age are more likely to maintain normal menstruation and fertility.

3. Pre-pregnancy counseling

As previously stated, a woman's fertility is not directly affected by SLE, since the ovaries are rarely impacted by the disease. Typically, it arises as a consequence of administered treatment, such as cyclophosphamide. The total administered dose of cyclophosphamide as well as the age of the administration, particularly in women over 35, have been proven to affect the risk of ovarian failure. Caution is warranted when administering follicular hormones, aiming at infertility treatment, due to the heightened risk of disease flare-ups and thrombosis in patients with antiphospholipid antibodies.

It is well advised that therapeutic approach to SLE begins before pregnancy, ensuring optimal health status at the onset of it. While the disease per se is not a contraindication for pregnancy, its potential complications, such as kidney failure or pulmonary hypertension should be taken into consideration. To minimize the risk of disease flare-ups during pregnancy, it is recommended that the disease remain inactive for at least 6 months prior to conception.

Administered medications must be deemed safe for pregnancy. These include prednisolone, azathioprine, cyclosporin A, and hydroxychloroquine, the latter of which has gained prominence recently and is considered a gold standard that may be administered throughout pregnancy.

In contrast, methotrexate and cyclophosphamide are teratogenic drugs, and their use should be discontinued at least 3 months before conception. Azathioprine is a recommended alternative. Classic non-steroidal anti-inflammatories (e.g., ibuprofen and diclofenac) are generally safe during pregnancy; however, they should be avoided after the 34th week of pregnancy due to the potential risk of premature closure of the fallopian tube. Newer non-steroidal anti-inflammatories such as cyclooxygenase-2 inhibitors should be avoided since their safety is compromised. Paracetamol and codeine analgesics are preferred analgesics and are often given in SLE. First-line treatment drugs in renal disease such as angiotensin converting enzyme (ACE) inhibitors and angiotensin II receptor antagonists are contraindicated and should not be used since they are linked to renal dysfunction. Thus, antihypertensive treatment in the context of SLE should include drugs safe for pregnancy, such as methyldopa-labitalol and nifedipine, the administration of which should begin before conception or in the initial stages of pregnancy. Assessment of pregnant SLE patients should start promptly and be monitored by a multidisciplinary team including an obstetrician-gynecologist, sonographer, rheumatologist, and midwife.

The frequency of visits depends on the individual's disease condition, but as a general recommendation, monthly visits are advised until the 28th week, followed by biweekly visits until week 36, and then weekly visits thereafter. Additionally, regular monitoring of fetal development is essential for all women, while Doppler assessment of the femoral arteries between the 20th and 24th week serves as a valuable indicator for predicting potential preeclampsia and intrauterine growth restriction (IUGR). Monitoring blood flow in the umbilical artery is also beneficial in cases of fetal IUGR.

It is important to note that the recording of fetal movements and cardiotocography remain reliable methods for monitoring fetal well-being. During pregnancy, levels of C3 and C4 fragments may elevate significantly compared to normal levels, while exacerbation of the disease with complement activation may occur even when C3 and C4 levels remain within normal ranges. In such cases, C3 and C4 levels can be low even in the absence of a disease flare-up. Conversely, if C3 and C4 levels increase by more than 25%, it likely indicates active disease. Thrombocytopenia, another indicator of disease activity, may also be observed in other situations connected to pregnancy, such as heparin therapy, preeclampsia, HELLP syndrome, and antiphospholipid syndrome. Consequently, monthly testing of complement and ds-DNA antibody levels is crucial, as well as a complete biochemical and hematological screening in conjunction with a urine test.

SLE often exhibits flare-ups during pregnancy and delivery, although they are mostly mild, and manifestations are limited to the skin. Exacerbation of the disease is associated with increased prematurity, while the nephritis observed appears to be an independent factor in fetal mortality. The treatment administered in cases of exanthema depends on the severity of the damage and the organs affected. In cases of arthritis, treatment options include non steroidal anti inflammatory drugs (NSAIDs), low doses of prednisolone (up to 10 mg/day) or hydroxychloroquine. Serositis usually responds to low doses of prednisolone. Other manifestations, such as renal damage, neuropsychiatric comorbidity, or other serious conditions, including cutaneous vasculitis, require more aggressive treatment. In these cases, higher doses of prednisolone are administered. However, the toxicity of steroids in pregnancy should not be neglected. For such reason, it is advisable to avoid high doses of steroids over prolonged periods. Early initiation of azathioprine is an ideal solution as it is well tolerated and has been utilized in many pregnant women with autoimmune conditions or transplanted organs. Some authors advocate for the intravenous administration of methylprednisolone; however, close monitoring of blood pressure and glucose levels is necessary in these instances. In general, women with SLE, uncomplicated by hypertension or irreversible renal damage prior to conception, experience a mild disease course during pregnancy. Moreover, pregnancy typically does not exacerbate renal disease. Instead, potentially pre-existing nephritis in lupus patients is an important risk factor for pregnant women. This group of women is at an elevated risk of miscarriage. An active disease 6 months before pregnancy is also an important prognostic indicator, while significant pre-existing non-reversible renal damage is associated with poor perinatal outcome [10]. When serum creatinine levels exceed 140 μmol/l, the likelihood of miscarriage rises to 50%, and when they surpass

	Normal	Preeclampsia	Lupus Nephritis
Blood pressure	Normal	High	Normal-high
Platelets	Normal	Low-normal	Low-normal
Complement	Normal	Normal-low	Low
Anti-ds-DNA	Normal-stable	Normal-stable	Increasing-high
Uric Acid	Normal	High	Normal
Creatinine	Normal	Normal-elevated	Normal-elevated
Hematuria	Absent	Possible	Present
Active urine sediment	No	No	Yes
Other SLE manifestations	No	No	Yes
Steroid response	No	No	Yes

Table 1.
Differential diagnosis of increasing proteinuria in pregnant women with SLE.

400 μmol/l, the percentage increases to 80%. Women with nephrotic syndrome require low-dose aspirin due to the increased risk of thrombosis, which should be administered through all stages of pregnancy, regardless of the potential existence of antiphospholipid antibodies. Women with pre-existing kidney disease should undergo at least monthly a 24-hour urine collection test, to assess factors such as creatinine clearance and proteinuria. Additionally, blood screening should be conducted to measure plasma creatinine levels, ds-DNA antibodies, and complement C3 and C4 levels. If proteinuria is detected during the urinalysis, the sample will undergo microscopic examination, in order to ascertain the presence of erythrocytes, which constitute evidence of active kidney disease. The differential diagnosis between SLE and normal pregnancy changes, as well as between active renal disease of SLE and preeclampsia, presents a frequent challenge for clinicians.

Sometimes, these conditions may coexist, and clinical laboratory monitoring may be a valuable asset on a case-by-case basis (refer to **Table 1**). Lupus nephritis is characterized by increased ds-DNA antibodies, decreased complement levels, clinical manifestations of organ involvement, and distinctive sediment in urine samples. In contrast, preeclampsia is characterized by increased levels of uric acid and liver enzymes, as well as non-specific sediment urine sample. Nevertheless, the distinction between lupus nephritis and preeclampsia is not always possible. In such cases, empirical treatment and monitoring of response are recommended, with kidney biopsy possibly required to guide therapeutic management. Corticosteroids are the treatment of choice.

4. Antiphospholipid syndrome

About 30–40% of women with SLE develop antiphospholipid antibodies, while a percentage of them have or are about to develop antiphospholipid syndrome (APS). The diagnosis of APS typically requires a history of thrombosis or recurrent pregnancy complications associated with antiphospholipid antibodies [11]. While APS is commonly observed in conjunction with SLE, it can also manifest as a primary condition or coexist with other connective tissue disorders. In particular, APS manifestations during pregnancy include recurrent miscarriages, IUGR, oligogamnio, preeclampsia, HELLP, placental abruption, and fetal death [12]. Obstetric history is an important aid in predicting future possible obstetric complications in the context of the disease. Approximately 50% of women with moderate to quite elevated levels of anticardiolipin IgG antibody (aCL) experience pregnancy loss, particularly those with a history of one fetal death. Conversely, slightly positive IgG aCL, as well as positive IgM or IgA antibodies, seem to be less associated with complications during pregnancy [12]. Placental infarctions are frequently observed; however, in some cases, placental damage may not be the sole cause of fetal distress. Aborted fetuses typically exhibit normal characteristics, although they may also test positive for aCL antibodies. However, neonatal complications do not appear to be directly attributed to these antibodies.

Few options exist concerning the treatment of pregnant women with antiphospholipid syndrome. Anticoagulant treatment is recommended as opposed to corticosteroids, which were previously more applicable in these cases [12]. Contemporary therapeutic approaches advocate for the use of aspirin, heparin, or a combination of both (**Table 2**). Two prospective studies reported that the administration of heparin combined with low-dose aspirin is more effective compared to aspirin alone in achieving live births in women with antiphospholipid syndrome and recurrent first-trimester miscarriages [13, 14]. These results were dismissed in another similar study [15]. In another study that involved women with positive antiphospholipid antibodies and regular miscarriages but a negative history of thrombosis or SLE, similar results (~80%) in live neonate births were observed after administration of either low-dose aspirin or placebo [16]. In conclusion, while the fact that ideal treatment for

Clinical picture	Recommended treatment
aPL positive women without a history of thrombosis or pregnancy loss risk	Low-dose aspirin (however, its efficacy has not been proven) due to minor toxicity.
Women with APS and previous first-trimester pregnancy loss	Low-dose aspirin. Recent studies suggest the addition of heparin, although the benefit beyond the 13th week. is not clear.
Women with APS and previous first or second-trimester pregnancy loss, IUGR, or placental abruption	Low-dose aspirin before conception with the addition of heparin subcutaneous (sbc) (dalteparin 5000 IU or enoxaparin 40 mg daily) after conception and throughout pregnancy.
Women with APS and previous venous thrombosis	These women are usually treated with anticoagulation per os. Since warfarin is contraindicated in the first trimester, a change should be made to aspirin plus heparin sbc (dalteparin 5000 IU or enoxaparin 40 mg daily). Doses will be doubled on the 16th to 20th week. In some cases anti-Xa levels measurement may be needed.
Women with APS and arterial thrombosis (especially with stroke)	If women develop neurological symptoms, the prophylactic dose of heparin sbc (dalteparin 5000 IU or enoxaparin 40 mg daily) should be increased in full anticoagulation. If the symptoms persist, re-introduce warfarin in the second trimester with a target INR of 2.5. Close monitoring is required in terms of anticoagulation to avoid fetal bleeding.
Women with APS and recurrent miscarriage despite proper anticoagulation	Treatment with iv immunoglobulin or even a low dose of prednisone with aspirin, heparin, or azathioprine. These approaches are currently experimental.

Table 2.
Recommended treatment in pregnant women with antiphospholipid syndrome (APS).

women with one or more pregnancy losses (second to third trimester) and a negative history of thrombosis remains controversial, most experts recommend the combination of heparin with low-dose aspirin [12].

Intravenous immunoglobulin (IVIG), in combination with heparin and low-dose aspirin, has also been given to women with a relevant obstetric history or pregnancy losses despite the use of heparin. However, a related study reported that additional administration of IVIG did not offer extra benefits compared to aspirin alone or heparin [17]. Warfarin should be administered cautiously in women with antiphospholipid syndrome and a history of thrombosis. If pregnancy is desired, the risk of fetal harm should be taken into account, especially between weeks 6 and 12 of pregnancy. These women should be switched to subcutaneous heparin as early as possible instead of warfarin. Some experts recommend this conversion before conception, while others advise it at the start of pregnancy. Heparin should be continued throughout pregnancy until warfarin can be resumed. Both medications are considered safe during breastfeeding.

4.1 Neonatal SLE

Neonatal SLE is associated with maternal anti-Ro and anti-La antibodies. It can appear in newborns of mothers with these antibodies, regardless of whether the mother exhibits clinical manifestations. The most common complication observed is congenital heart block at a rate of 2%, with a recurrence rate of 16% in subsequent pregnancies. Neonatal SLE has a mortality rate of 24%, and approximately 50% of surviving infants will require a pacemaker within the first year of life. Once detected, the block can no longer be reversed; however, in some cases, a second-degree block has been converted to first-degree after administering dexamethasone. In cases of hydrops fetalis development, dexamethasone, salbutamol, or digoxin may be administered, taking into account the possible maternal risks. To prevent another fetal heart block in women with a history, some researchers recommend IVIG administration between the 12th and 24th week of gestation. Neonatal SLE presents similarly to adult-onset SLE, often following exposure to the sun or UV radiation within the first 2 weeks of life. It typically resolves within 6 months. Topical steroids can be used as treatment. Other rarer manifestations of neonatal SLE include abnormal liver function tests and thrombocytopenia, which typically regress after the first year.

5. SLE and gynecological cancers

Several significant rheumatic disorders are linked to an elevated likelihood of developing different types of cancers [18]. There has been a growing interest in investigating connections between autoimmune disorders, such as SLE, and the risk of cancer, while there are a number of studies that have explored the potential risks associated with SLE. Current data suggests a slight (10–15%) increase in overall cancer risk in individuals with SLE compared to the general population [19].

A large multisite cohort study by Bernatsky et al., involving 30 centers and 16,409 patients who were observed for 121,283 person-years, found a standardized incidence ratio (SIR) of 1.14 (95% confidence interval (CI): 1.05–1.23) in the overall incidence of malignancy. The most noticeable increased risk was observed in hematologic cancers (SIR: 3.02, 95%, CI: 2.48–3.63), particularly non-Hodgkin lymphoma (NHL)

(SIR: 4.39, 95% CI: 3.46–5.49). Other cancers suggested to have an increased risk were lung (SIR: 1.30, 95% CI: 1.04–1.60) and hepatobiliary cancers (SIR: 1.87, 95% CI: 0.97–3.27) [20]. Similar results have been reported in two more studies with a large number of patients. The first cohort involved 30,478 SLE patients who were observed for 157.969 person-years and found an increased overall cancer risk (SIR: 1.14, 95% CI: 1.07–1.20) [21]. The second study which followed 11,763 SLE patients between 1996 and 2007, also found an increased risk of cancer (SIR: 1.76 95% CI: 1.74–1.79) [22]. Conversely, individuals with SLE may have a reduced risk for certain cancers, such as breast, prostate, and other cancers [19, 20].

Due to SLE being primarily a disease affecting women, there is a special interest in the occurrence of cancers in the female genital tract. These malignancies include cancers of the vulva, cervical, ovarian, and endometrial cancers. As far as the incidence of gynecological malignancies for people with SLE is concerned, existing data seems controversial [23].

With current data remaining inconclusive, several studies seem to have found a negative correlation between ovarian cancer and SLE [23–25]. It should be taken into account that ovarian cancer in SLE patients is rare and may compromise the validity of any results. In a study of 5715 hospitalized SLE patients, the SIR for ovarian cancer was 0.48 (95% CI, 0.19–0.99) [26]. On the other hand, one report suggested an increase of ovarian cancer in patients with cutaneous lupus erythematosus (two- to fourfold increased only in cutaneous lupus and not SLE) [27], and within the first 3 years of the diagnosis of SLE [28]. Finally, Song et al. in a meta-analysis of 24 studies found that 11 studies failed to display any vital association between SLE and ovarian cancer (pooled SIR: 0.92, 95% CI: 0.74–1.33, P: 0.309, I 2 = 14.2%) [29]. The cause of this low incidence of ovarian cancer among SLE patients remains unclear. Individuals with SLE have a smaller risk for various hormone-sensitive cancers (such as breast and endometrial cancer). This could suggest a link between SLE and an altered metabolism of estrogen and/or other hormones [30]. An unproven hypothesis is that SLE patients tend to have a higher age at menarche and a lower age at menopause compared to the general population, resulting in a generally reduced exposure to endogenous estrogens [23]. Furthermore, it has been suggested that the observed low rates of ovarian cancers in SLE patients may be linked to certain lupus autoantibodies [31].

Several studies have suggested that SLE may have a protective effect on the risk of endometrial cancer [23, 25]. Bernatsky's international, multisite prospective, cohort study showed that SLE patients have a decreased risk of endometrial cancer SIR: 0.44, 95% (CI: 0.23–0.77) [20]. In addition, a meta-analysis of five large SLE cohorts involving 47,325 SLE patients being observed for a total of 282,553 person-years strongly reported an SIR of 0.7195%(CI: 0.55–0.91) [25]. This seems to contradict Song's meta-analysis of six studies that did not manage to show any correlation between endometrial cancer and SLE (pooled SIR =0.70, 95% CI = 0.46–1.07, P = 0.035, I 2 = 58.3%) [32]. Similar to ovarian cancer, the precise biological mechanism through which SLE might reduce the risk of endometrial cancer remains unclear. There are several possible theories. It has been shown that patients with SLE exhibit higher levels of sex hormone-binding globulin (SHBG). This leads to decreased levels of bioavailable estrogen, potentially lowering the risk of endometrial cancer and other hormone-sensitive cancers. Furthermore, circulating autoantibodies that target host DNA, a characteristic of SLE, such as 3E10, seem to be harmful to tumors and cancer cells with defective homologous recombination repair, similar to some ovarian and endometrial cancers [32].

Interestingly, a strong correlation between SLE and increased risk for vulvar, vaginal and anal cancers has been found [23]. Bernatsky's cohort study identified a notable increase in the risk of vulvar (SIR: 3.78; 95% CI: 1.52–7.78) and vaginal carcinoma (SIR: 3.80; 95% CI: 0.46–13.74) [20]. Similarly, Song, in his meta-analysis, found eight studies that revealed an increased risk of vagina/vulva cancers (pooled SIR: 3.48, 95% CI: 2.69–4.50, P: 0.813, I 2: 0.0%) [29]. However, it is important to always consider the low absolute number of these rare malignancies when interpreting the results.

Reports regarding the incidence of cervical cancer in patients with SLE are conflicting [20, 21, 23, 29]. Cervical dysplasia, the precursor to cervical cancer, has been shown to be more prevalent in individuals with SLE compared to the general population (OR: 8.66; 95% CI: 3.75–20.00) [33, 34]. While the majority of low-grade cervical intraepithelial neoplasia (CIN) lesions tend to regress spontaneously, most high-grade cervical dysplasia, specifically CIN 2 or 3, does not. Persistent human papillomavirus (HPV) infection, a significant risk factor for cervical cancer, is associated with various factors including HPV genotype, older age, coexisting infections, immunosuppression, and inflammation [35]. Despite the large number of studies that have found an elevated risk of cervical dysplasia in patients with SLE, it remains unclear whether there is an increased risk of actual invasive cervical cancer. For example, a study of Swedish registers that matched 4976 patients with SLE with 29,703 other women found that there was an increased risk of CIN 1 (HR: 2.33; 95% CI: 1.58–3.44), CIN 2–3 (HR: 1.95; 95% CI: 1.43–2.65) and any CIN (HR: 2.12; 95% CI: 1.65–2.71), but not an increase in invasive cervical cancer (HR: 1.64; 95%CI: 0.54–5.02) [36]. In this study, all invasive cervical cancers were observed in patients treated with immunosuppressives. There are other studies in agreement with the same correlation between CIN and invasive cervical cancer [19, 21, 23]. In contrast, there are papers that support the increase not only in CIN but also in invasive cervical cancer [37, 38]. For instance, Song et al. in their meta-analysis found a 50% increased risk of cervical cancer. In 11 studies that SLE was related to increased risk of cervix cancers (pooled SIR: 1.56, 95% CI: 1.29–1.88, P: 0.404, I 2 = 4.1%) [29].

Bias in the studies presented or included in the meta-analysis, whether prospective or retrospective, the small number of patients with invasive cancer, problems in reporting, discrepancies in screening, short follow-up times, the severity of the autoimmune disease, coexisting factors, and other methodological differences may explain the aforementioned differences.

In the case of cervical, vulvar, and vaginal cancers, there is a strong association with HPV infection. Cervical cancer is the most common HPV-related disease [39]. There is evidence of an increased rate of HPV infection among women with SLE and infections with high-risk aggressive variants at a high viral load [40, 41]. A Korean study with 134 SLE patients showed that SLE itself was an independent risk factor for high-risk HPV infection, with SLE patients having greater prevalence of high-risk HPV infection (24.6% vs. 7.9%, P < 0.001, OR: 3.8, 95% CI: 2.5–5.7) and of abnormal cervical cytology results (16.4 vs. 2.8%, P < 0.001, OR: 4.4, 95% CI 2.5–7.8) compared with controls [42]. Innate autoimmune defects and/or immunosuppression may result in the inability of the immune system to clear the virus. Poor HPV clearance may result in the development of CIN [23, 43]. For patients with SLE, it is not known whether this could be attributed to baseline defective immunity to HPV or secondary to medication exposure.

A growing interest in immunosuppressive therapy as a potential factor contributing to increased cancer risk in patients with autoimmune diseases has also been observed. There have been several attempts to answer the question of whether iatrogenic immunosuppression increases cancer risk in patients with SLE, presenting mixed results. There are studies suggesting that the risk of high-grade cervical dysplasia of cervical cancer is the same for patients with SLE irrespective of the use of systemic immunosuppressants [38, 40]. One study found a higher incidence of cervical cancer, even in women with SLE who have never used immunosuppressants [37]. However, in this study, the relatively low frequency of exposure to immunosuppressants, combined with the rare occurrence of cancer within the cohort, make the interpretation of the actual impact difficult. Interestingly, other studies showed the exact opposite results. One study suggested that long-term use of immunosuppression doubled the prevalence of low-grade and high-grade intraepithelial lesions [43]. There are studies that even suggest the dose-dependent correlation between the immunosuppressive drug and the likelihood of the patient developing cancer [44, 45].

It is essential to acknowledge the potential presence of confounding factors. There may be other factors related to treatment, severity of the disease and indications of treatment that might explain some associations. One of the difficulties in interpreting these results lies in the fact that patients with SLE receiving potent immunosuppressive therapies, especially cyclophosphamide, probably have higher disease activity. Even though there are a few small studies denying the relation between disease severity and risk for CIN in patients with SLE, there is not enough evidence to suggest that a higher disease burden is related to a lower or higher risk of cancer [46].

A notable study in Denmark found that individuals with autoimmune disorders did not show an increased risk of developing cervical cancer. Furthermore, the study indicated that the utilization of immunosuppressants generally did not correlate with heightened risk, with the exception of azathioprine use [47].

Moreover, there are papers that suggest that despite treatment with immunosuppressive therapies like cyclophosphamide, methotrexate, azathioprine, and mycophenolate mofetil, these patients may be at higher risk of developing cervical neoplasia, while those treated with antimalarials are not [36, 48]. In addition to this, there are indications that antimalarial drugs such as hydroxychloroquine may play a protective role against cancer in patients diagnosed with SLE [48]. However, at present, there is not sufficient evidence to support that claim. The same applies to the use of aspirin and non-steroidal anti-inflammatory drugs, which have been linked with a decreased risk of some cancers but not in patients with SLE [49].

Screening for cancers is important in the entire population. Generally, there are no well-established guidelines for ovarian, uterine, and vulvar cancers, but there are for cervical cancer. Due to the suggestion of increased CIN and cervical cancer risk, cervical cancer screening is particularly important for patients with SLE. Screening for cervical cancer might help in screening the rarer vulvar and vaginal cancers that have a higher incidence in patients with SLE, especially given the fact that women are not very familiar with and informed about other HPV-related cancers [50].

It could be suggested that since patients with SLE have regular follow-ups for their autoimmune disease, they might get more screening testing for cancer. On the other hand, due to both the nature of SLE and the fact that SLE patients seek care from specialists who are experts on autoimmune diseases and not cancer, screening for other diseases might be overlooked. There are studies showing similar participation of women with SLE and controls in screening programs for cervical cancer [47, 51]. A prospective study revealed that the proportion of younger women with SLE attending a screening visit was lower, but the difference was relatively small [36]. Nevertheless, other studies have suggested that women with SLE are less likely to undergo the recommended screening for cervical cancer compared to the general population (33% versus 56%) [52]. About half of the SLE patients are not up to date in their screening schedule [53]. Only 9 of 27 patients with SLE aged less than 30 years old had a cytology test in the previous 12 months (33%, 95% CI: 19–52). Race and education level appear to be related to the screening rate. Women with more severe disease (based on SLE/ACR damage index scores) were the least likely to have undergone cervical screening.

SLE specialists should encourage all their patients, especially those with a history of dysplasia, not to overlook their cancer screening appointments.

There are no original research studies comparing cancer screening strategies for patients with SLE. Tessier-Cloutier et al. published a systematic review on cancer screening specifically for patients with SLE [54]. Among the 79 original research papers, 25 gave screening recommendations, of which 14 proposed additional cancer screening, while 11 advocated adherence to the general population screening programs. Some articles suggested annual screening for cervical cancer and testing for HPV in patients who had received cyclophosphamide in the past.

A recent publication regarding guidelines for cervical cancer screening in immunosuppressed women without HIV infection proposed that due to the elevated risk of cervical intraepithelial neoplasia (CIN), women with systemic lupus erythematosus (SLE) should adhere to the same screening protocols as women with HIV, irrespective of whether they are receiving immunosuppressant treatments or not [55].

Their recommendations include:

- Cytology before the age of 30 years old.

- Co-testing after the age of 30 years old. Cytology could be acceptable. In case of using only cytology, it should be performed annually. If three consecutive cytology results are normal, cytology could be performed every 3 years.

- When using co-testing, there should be a baseline co-test of HPV with cytology. If the HPV is negative and the cytology normal, co-testing could be performed every 3 years.

- If the patient had immunosuppressant therapy before the age of 21 years old, screening should begin within 1 year of the first sexual encounter.

- Screening should be continued throughout lifetime.

- Screening could discontinue based on shared discussion regarding quality and duration of life rather than age.

The European League Against Rheumatism (EULAR) recommends that women with SLE should undergo screening for malignancies as the general population (level of agreement D) and that women who are heavily immunosuppressed should be monitored with vigilance (level of agreement B) with the suggested timing for cytology examination to be once a year [56].

Vaccines are one of the most effective tools to prevent infectious diseases. In the last two decades, three non-live protein subunit vaccines for HPV have been approved [57]. The bivalent (bHPV – aimed against serotypes 16 and 18), the quadrivalent (qHPV – against serotypes 6, 11, 16, and 18), and most recently, the 9-valent (9vHPV – against serotypes 6, 11, 16, 18, 31, 33,45, 52, and 58).

Admittedly, there are several concerns about vaccination in immunocompromised patients. Some of these concerns include the potential risk of exacerbation of the underlying disease, the possibility that a live-attenuated vaccine may induce an overt infection, and that the vaccine will not be effective and immunogenic since it cannot induce both adequate antibody levels and the memory to achieve short term and long-term protection [58].

Overall, immunosuppressive drugs typically do not appear to impair the effectiveness of vaccines [59, 60]. However, rituximab, an anti-CD-20 antibody, stands as an exception as it can impact immune responses to vaccines. It is advised that vaccination should take place at least 6 months after rituximab administration [58].

Even though the immune response generated from a vaccine against HPV may be lower in patients with SLE compared to the general population, studies suggest that it is safe and effective in individuals with autoimmune diseases, including SLE [59, 61].

A case-control study of 50 patients with SLE between the ages of 18 and 35 years old who were vaccinated with the quadrivalent HPV vaccine found that the seroconversion rates of antibodies to HPV serotypes 6, 11, 16, and 18 at 7 and 12 months were similar between the SLE patients and the control group [62]. Specifically, at month 7, the seroconversion rates of anti-HPV types 6, 11, 16, and 18 in patients with SLE and controls were 74%, 76%, 92%, 76% and 96%, 95%, 98%, and 93%, respectively. At month 12, the seroconversion rates in patients with SLE and controls were 82%, 89%, 95%, 76%, 98%, 98%, 98%, and 80%, respectively. Apart from antibody titers for type HPV-6, both at 7 and 12 months being lower in SLE patients, the other antibody titers did not statistically differ. Patients did have a lower specific immune response when compared to the control group, but most of them produced protective antibody levels. A considerable number of patients were receiving immunosuppressive medications. No significant differences in the seroconversion rates were observed between patients receiving treatment and those who were not. No significant difference was reported between patients who were on various medications, except for those who were taking mycophenolate mofetil. The most common adverse event was erythema and pain at the injection site that subsided spontaneously after 1–2 days. Crucially, no difference was observed in disease flares nor significant changes in the titers of serologic autoimmune markers [62].

The researchers examined the same patients 5 years later and found out that immunogenicity of the vaccine was retained in most of them. The levels of antibody titers to HPV-6 and 16 were significantly lower in patients than controls, and there were 7 (21%) SLE patients with seroreversion in at least 1 anti-HPV antibody. The latter had significantly more disease flares and needed higher doses of immunosuppressive medications [63]. Repeating HPV vaccinations for those patients could be considered, but there is no evidence about the safety and efficacy of this practice.

Certain case reports and case series have expressed concern regarding the use of HPV vaccines, as they identified a potential association with the onset of autoimmune diseases [64]. Although, population-based studies consistently demonstrate that HPV vaccines are not linked to an increased incidence of new-onset autoimmune diseases [65].

EULAR recommends that all patients with SLE should be vaccinated against HPV according to the recommendations for the general population (strength of recommendation C) [60]. The US Centers for Disease Control and Prevention (CDC) recommends the vaccine for any immunocompromised patients up to age of 26 years old [66].

In general, cancer is an important cause of morbidity and mortality for SLE patients. Patients with SLE have an increased risk of cancers, especially NHL and lung cancer. As far as gynecological cancers are concerned, there is an increased risk for cancers of the vulva and the vagina, whereas there seems to be a protective correlation for ovarian and uterine cancers. Even though there are conflicting reports about cervical cancer, there is a definite connection between SLE, HPV infections, and CIN. Both family doctors and specialists should encourage their patients to follow cancer screening programs, undergo vaccination where it is appropriate, and try to minimize other known cancer risk factors (such as smoking and obesity).

6. Conclusion

With advancements in the diagnosis and treatment of patients with SLE, the prognosis has improved during the last few years. Thus, successful pregnancy outcomes are now more attainable than ever before. However, significant morbidity still exists for both the mother and her fetus. Early counseling prior to conception, vigilant and continuous monitoring of the patient, and collaboration among specialists are essential for achieving the best perinatal outcomes. In general, pregnancies complicated by SLE carry a higher risk of spontaneous abortions, preeclampsia, IUGR, fetal death, and preterm birth. The magnitude of risk depends on the presence or absence of complications lupus nephritis, hypertension, antiphospholipid antibodies and pericarditis. Women with SLE usually require treatment that may complicate the pregnancy. Therefore, having the appropriate therapeutic approach before and after pregnancy is crucial for achieving optimal perinatal outcomes. Up to date, corticosteroids have been used extensively and safely during pregnancy. Corticosteroids have been extensively and safely used during pregnancy. Additionally, hydroxychloroquine and azathioprine have demonstrated efficacy with no observed increased risk of congenital anomalies, unlike methotrexate and cyclophosphamide, which are contraindicated in pregnancy (**Table 3**). Antithrombotic drugs also improve the perinatal outcomes in cases of

---

- Pregnancy can alter the activity of SLE and increase the risk of thrombotic episodes.
- SLE and antiphospholipid syndrome increase the possibility of miscarriage, intrauterine delayed development, and premature birth.
- Pregnancy should be planned at least 6 months after the last exacerbation of the disease.
- Hydroxychloroquine should not be discontinued at the beginning of pregnancy since a flare-up may be triggered.
- SLE should be carefully regulated throughout pregnancy. Corticosteroids are the drugs of choice.
- Congenital heart diseases are closely associated with the presence of anti-Ro/anti-La antibodies in the mother.
- Aspirin and heparin are the drugs of choice in the prevention of miscarriage in antiphospholipid syndrome.
- Regular obstetric and medical monitoring by experienced staff throughout the pregnancy increases the probability of a successful pregnancy outcome.

Table 3.
Practical issues.

antiphospholipid syndrome. Finally, a rare condition of fetal heart block has been associated with the presence of anti-Ro and anti-La antibodies in the mother.

Later in the woman's life, SLE patients have an increased risk for gynecological cancers, especially cervical cancer. The immune suppression related to the regimens that the patient receives or even the immune dysregulation that SLE heralds renders the patient a predisposition for any type of malignancy. Cyclophosphamide is well known to be related to bladder cancer and other cancers as well. Vigilance and meticulous GYn examination is warranted for SLE patients.

Author details

Ismini Anagnostaki[1], Konstantinos Zacharis[1], Konstantia Loga[2] and
Ioannis Gkougkourelas[3*]

1 Gynecology and Obstretics Clinic, General Hospital of Lamia, Lamia, Greece

2 Department of Medical Oncology, School of Medicine Aristotle University of Thessaloniki, Thessaloniki, Greece

3 Internal Medicine Clinic General Hospital of Thessaloniki "Agios Dimitrios", Thessaloniki, Greece

*Address all correspondence to: igkougkourelas@gmail.com

IntechOpen

References

[1] Hickman RA, Gordon C. Causes and management of infertility in systemic lupus erythematosus. Rheumatology (Oxford, England). 2011;**50**(9):1551-1558

[2] Hamouda RK, Arzoun H, Sahib I, Escudero Mendez L, Srinivasan M, Shoukrie SI, et al. The comorbidity of endometriosis and systemic lupus erythematosus: A systematic review. Cureus. 2023;**15**(7):e42362

[3] Kunzler ALF, Tsokos GC. Infections in patients with systemic lupus erythematosus: The contribution of primary immune defects versus treatment-induced immunosuppression. European Journal of Rheumatology. 2023;**10**(4):148-158

[4] Boumpas DT, Austin HA 3rd, Vaughan EM, Yarboro CH, Klippel JH, Balow JE. Risk for sustained amenorrhea in patients with systemic lupus erythematosus receiving intermittent pulse cyclophosphamide therapy. Annals of Internal Medicine. 1993;**119**(5):366-369

[5] Mok CC, Lau CS, Wong RW. Risk factors for ovarian failure in patients with systemic lupus erythematosus receiving cyclophosphamide therapy. Arthritis and Rheumatism. 1998;**41**(5):831-837

[6] McDermott EM, Powell RJ. Incidence of ovarian failure in systemic lupus erythematosus after treatment with pulse cyclophosphamide. Annals of the Rheumatic Diseases. 1996;**55**(4):224-229

[7] Park MC, Park YB, Jung SY, Chung IH, Choi KH, Lee SK. Risk of ovarian failure and pregnancy outcome in patients with lupus nephritis treated with intravenous cyclophosphamide pulse therapy. Lupus. 2004;**13**(8):569-574

[8] Langevitz P, Klein L, Pras M, Many A. The effect of cyclophosphamide pulses on fertility in patients with lupus nephritis. American Journal of Reproductive Immunology. 1992;**28**(3-4):157-158

[9] Ioannidis JP, Katsifis GE, Tzioufas AG, Moutsopoulos HM. Predictors of sustained amenorrhea from pulsed intravenous cyclophosphamide in premenopausal women with systemic lupus erythematosus. The Journal of Rheumatology. 2002;**29**(10):2129-2135

[10] Oviasu E, Hicks J, Cameron JS. The outcome of pregnancy in women with lupus nephritis. Lupus. 1991;**1**(1):19-25

[11] Miyakis S, Lockshin MD, Atsumi T, Branch DW, Brey RL, Cervera R, et al. International consensus statement on an update of the classification criteria for definite antiphospholipid syndrome (APS). Journal of Thrombosis and Haemostasis. 2006;**4**(2):295-306

[12] Di Prima FA, Valenti O, Hyseni E, Giorgio E, Faraci M, Renda E, et al. Antiphospholipid Syndrome during pregnancy: the state of the art. Journal of Prenatal Medicine. 2011;**5**(2):41-53

[13] Rai R, Cohen H, Dave M, Regan L. Randomised controlled trial of aspirin and aspirin plus heparin in pregnant women with recurrent miscarriage associated with phospholipid antibodies (or antiphospholipid antibodies). BMJ. 1997;**314**(7076):253-257

[14] Kutteh WH. Antiphospholipid antibody-associated recurrent pregnancy loss: treatment with heparin and low-dose aspirin is superior to low-dose aspirin alone. American Journal of Obstetrics and Gynecology. 1996;**174**(5):1584-1589

[15] Farquharson RG, Quenby S, Greaves M. Antiphospholipid syndrome in pregnancy: a randomized, controlled trial of treatment. Obstetrics and Gynecology. 2002;**100**(3):408-413

[16] Pattison NS, Chamley LW, Birdsall M, Zanderigo AM, Liddell HS, McDougall J. Does aspirin have a role in improving pregnancy outcome for women with the antiphospholipid syndrome? A randomized controlled trial. American Journal of Obstetrics and Gynecology. 2000;**183**(4):1008-1012

[17] Branch DW, Peaceman AM, Druzin M, Silver RK, El-Sayed Y, Silver RM, et al. A multicenter, placebo-controlled pilot study of intravenous immune globulin treatment of antiphospholipid syndrome during pregnancy. The Pregnancy Loss Study Group. American Journal of Obstetrics and Gynecology. 2000;**182**(1 Pt 1): 122-127

[18] Egiziano G, Bernatsky S, Shah AA. Cancer and autoimmunity: Harnessing longitudinal cohorts to probe the link. Best Practice & Research. Clinical Rheumatology. 2016;**30**(1):53-62

[19] Bernatsky S, Boivin JF, Joseph L, Rajan R, Zoma A, Manzi S, et al. An international cohort study of cancer in systemic lupus erythematosus. Arthritis and Rheumatism. 2005;**52**(5):1481-1490

[20] Bernatsky S, Ramsey-Goldman R, Urowitz MB, Hanly JG, Gordon C, Petri MA, et al. Cancer risk in a large inception systemic lupus erythematosus cohort: Effects of demographic characteristics, smoking, and medications. Arthritis Care & Research (Hoboken). 2021;**73**(12):1789-1795

[21] Parikh-Patel A, White RH, Allen M, Cress R. Cancer risk in a cohort of patients with systemic lupus erythematosus (SLE) in California. Cancer Causes & Control. 2008;**19**(8):887-894

[22] Chen YJ, Chang YT, Wang CB, Wu CY. Malignancy in systemic lupus erythematosus: a nationwide cohort study in Taiwan. The American Journal of Medicine. 2010;**123**(12):1150.e1-1150.e6

[23] Ladouceur A, Tessier-Cloutier B, Clarke AE, Ramsey-Goldman R, Gordon C, Hansen JE, et al. Cancer and systemic lupus erythematosus. Rheumatic Diseases Clinics of North America. 2020;**46**(3):533-550

[24] Cao L, Tong H, Xu G, Liu P, Meng H, Wang J, et al. Systemic lupus erythematous and malignancy risk: a meta-analysis. PLoS One. 2015;**10**(4):e0122964

[25] Bernatsky S, Ramsey-Goldman R, Foulkes WD, Gordon C, Clarke AE. Breast, ovarian, and endometrial malignancies in systemic lupus erythematosus: a meta-analysis. British Journal of Cancer. 2011;**104**(9):1478-1481

[26] Björnådal L, Löfström B, Yin L, Lundberg IE, Ekbom A. Increased cancer incidence in a Swedish cohort of patients with systemic lupus erythematosus. Scandinavian Journal of Rheumatology. 2002;**31**(2):66-71

[27] Westermann R, Zobbe K, Cordtz R, Haugaard JH, Dreyer L. Increased cancer risk in patients with cutaneous lupus erythematosus and systemic lupus erythematosus compared with the general population: A Danish nationwide cohort study. Lupus. 2021;**30**(5):752-761

[28] Zhou Z, Liu H, Yang Y, Zhou J, Zhao L, Chen H, et al. The five major autoimmune diseases increase the risk of cancer: epidemiological data from

a large-scale cohort study in China. Cancer Communications (Lond). 2022;**42**(5):435-446

[29] Song L, Wang Y, Zhang J, Song N, Xu X, Lu Y. The risks of cancer development in systemic lupus erythematosus (SLE) patients: a systematic review and meta-analysis. Arthritis Research & Therapy. 2018;**20**(1):270

[30] Yagita M, Hata S, Miyata H, Kakita H, Tsukamoto T, Muso E, et al. Systemic lupus erythematosus associated with ovarian cancer. Internal Medicine. 2019;**58**(5):731-735

[31] Hansen JE, Chan G, Liu Y, Hegan DC, Dalal S, Dray E, et al. Targeting cancer with a lupus autoantibody. Science Translational Medicine. 2012;**4**(157):157ra42

[32] Wan A, Zhao WD, Tao JH. Causal effects of systemic lupus erythematosus on endometrial cancer: A univariable and multivariable Mendelian randomization study. Frontiers in Oncology. 2022;**12**:930243

[33] Chen Y, Wu X, Liu L. Association between systemic lupus erythematosus and risk of cervical atypia: A meta-analysis. Lupus. 2021;**30**(13):2075-2088

[34] Zard E, Arnaud L, Mathian A, Chakhtoura Z, Hie M, Touraine P, et al. Increased risk of high grade cervical squamous intraepithelial lesions in systemic lupus erythematosus: A meta-analysis of the literature. Autoimmunity Reviews. 2014;**13**(7):730-735

[35] Wheeler CM. Natural history of human papillomavirus infections, cytologic and histologic abnormalities, and cancer. Obstetrics and Gynecology Clinics of North America. 2008;**35**(4):519-536 vii

[36] Wadström H, Arkema EV, Sjöwall C, Askling J, Simard JF. Cervical neoplasia in systemic lupus erythematosus: a nationwide study. Rheumatology (Oxford, England). 2017;**56**(4):613-619

[37] Cibere J, Sibley J, Haga M. Systemic lupus erythematosus and the risk of malignancy. Lupus. 2001;**10**(6):394-400

[38] Kim SC, Glynn RJ, Giovannucci E, Hernández-Díaz S, Liu J, Feldman S, et al. Risk of high-grade cervical dysplasia and cervical cancer in women with systemic inflammatory diseases: a population-based cohort study. Annals of the Rheumatic Diseases. 2015;**74**(7):1360-1367

[39] Okunade KS. Human papillomavirus and cervical cancer. Journal of Obstetrics and Gynaecology. 2020;**40**(5):602-608

[40] Lyrio LD, Grassi MF, Santana IU, Olavarria VG, Gomes Ado N, Costa Pinto L, et al. Prevalence of cervical human papillomavirus infection in women with systemic lupus erythematosus. Rheumatology International. 2013;**33**(2):335-340

[41] Nath R, Mant C, Luxton J, Hughes G, Raju KS, Shepherd P, et al. High risk of human papillomavirus type 16 infections and of development of cervical squamous intraepithelial lesions in systemic lupus erythematosus patients. Arthritis and Rheumatism. 2007;**57**(4):619-625

[42] Lee YH, Choe JY, Park SH, Park YW, Lee SS, Kang YM, et al. Prevalence of human papilloma virus infections and cervical cytological abnormalities among Korean women with systemic lupus erythematosus. Journal of Korean Medical Science. 2010;**25**(10):1431-1437

[43] Klumb EM, Araújo ML Jr, Jesus GR, Santos DB, Oliveira AV,

Albuquerque EM, et al. Is higher prevalence of cervical intraepithelial neoplasia in women with lupus due to immunosuppression? Journal of Clinical Rheumatology. 2010;**16**(4):153-157

[44] Ognenovski VM, Marder W, Somers EC, Johnston CM, Farrehi JG, Selvaggi SM, et al. Increased incidence of cervical intraepithelial neoplasia in women with systemic lupus erythematosus treated with intravenous cyclophosphamide. The Journal of Rheumatology. 2004;**31**(9):1763-1767

[45] Bernatsky S, Ramsey-Goldman R, Gordon C, Joseph L, Boivin JF, Rajan R, et al. Factors associated with abnormal Pap results in systemic lupus erythematosus. Rheumatology (Oxford, England). 2004;**43**(11):1386-1389

[46] Dhar JP, Gregoire L, Lancaster W, Stark A, Schwartz AG, Schultz D, et al. Risk for cervical intraepithelial neoplasia in systemic lupus erythematosus is not related to disease severity. Current Rheumatology Reviews. 2013;**9**(4):301-304

[47] Dugué PA, Rebolj M, Hallas J, Garred P, Lynge E. Risk of cervical cancer in women with autoimmune diseases, in relation with their use of immunosuppressants and screening: population-based cohort study. International Journal of Cancer. 2015;**136**(6):E711-E719

[48] Ruiz-Irastorza G, Ugarte A, Egurbide MV, Garmendia M, Pijoan JI, Martinez-Berriotxoa A, et al. Antimalarials may influence the risk of malignancy in systemic lupus erythematosus. Annals of the Rheumatic Diseases. 2007;**66**(6):815-817

[49] Tessier-Cloutier B, Clarke AE, Ramsey-Goldman R, Gordon C, Hansen JE, Bernatsky S. Systemic lupus erythematosus and malignancies: a review article. Rheumatic Diseases Clinics of North America. 2014;**40**(3):497-506 viii

[50] Dhar JP, Walline H, Mor G, Fathallah L, Szpunar S, Saravolatz L, et al. Cervical health in systemic lupus erythematosus. Women's Health Reports (New Rochelle). 2023;**4**(1):328-337

[51] Bruera S, Lei X, Zogala R, Pundole X, Zhao H, Giordano SH, et al. Cervical cancer screening in women with systemic lupus erythematosus. Arthritis Care & Research (Hoboken). 2021;**73**(12):1796-1803

[52] Bernatsky SR, Cooper GS, Mill C, Ramsey-Goldman R, Clarke AE, Pineau CA. Cancer screening in patients with systemic lupus erythematosus. The Journal of Rheumatology. 2006;**33**(1):45-49

[53] Chung SH, Oshima K, Singleton M, Thomason J, Currier C, McCartney S, et al. Determinants of cervical cancer screening patterns among women with systemic lupus erythematosus. The Journal of Rheumatology. 2022;**49**(11):1236-1241

[54] Tessier-Cloutier B, Clarke AE, Pineau CA, Keeling S, Bissonauth A, Ramsey-Goldman R, et al. What investigations are needed to optimally monitor for malignancies in SLE? Lupus. 2015;**24**(8):781-787

[55] Moscicki AB, Flowers L, Huchko MJ, Long ME, MacLaughlin KL, Murphy J, et al. Guidelines for cervical cancer screening in immunosuppressed women without HIV infection. Journal of Lower Genital Tract Disease. 2019;**23**(2):87-101

[56] Andreoli L, Bertsias GK, Agmon-Levin N, Brown S, Cervera R, Costedoat-Chalumeau N, et al.

EULAR recommendations for women's health and the management of family planning, assisted reproduction, pregnancy and menopause in patients with systemic lupus erythematosus and/or antiphospholipid syndrome. Annals of the Rheumatic Diseases. 2017;**76**(3):476-485

[57] Pils S, Joura EA. From the monovalent to the nine-valent HPV vaccine. Clinical Microbiology and Infection. 2015;**21**(9):827-833

[58] Grein IHR, Groot N, Lacerda MI, Wulffraat N, Pileggi G. HPV infection and vaccination in Systemic Lupus Erythematosus patients: what we really should know. Pediatric Rheumatology. 2016;**14**(1):12

[59] Heijstek MW, Ott de Bruin LM, Borrow R, van der Klis F, Koné-Paut I, Fasth A, et al. Vaccination in paediatric patients with auto-immune rheumatic diseases: a systemic literature review for the European League against Rheumatism evidence-based recommendations. Autoimmunity Reviews. 2011;**11**(2):112-122

[60] Furer V, Rondaan C, Heijstek MW, Agmon-Levin N, van Assen S, Bijl M, et al. 2019 update of EULAR recommendations for vaccination in adult patients with autoimmune inflammatory rheumatic diseases. Annals of the Rheumatic Diseases. 2020;**79**(1):39-52

[61] Dhar JP, Essenmacher L, Dhar R, Magee A, Ager J, Sokol RJ. The safety and immunogenicity of quadrivalent HPV (qHPV) vaccine in systemic lupus erythematosus. Vaccine. 2017;**35**(20):2642-2646

[62] Mok CC, Ho LY, Fong LS, To CH. Immunogenicity and safety of a quadrivalent human papillomavirus

vaccine in patients with systemic lupus erythematosus: a case-control study. Annals of the Rheumatic Diseases. 2013;**72**(5):659-664

[63] Mok CC, Ho LY, To CH. Long-term immunogenicity of a quadrivalent human papillomavirus vaccine in systemic lupus erythematosus. Vaccine. 2018;**36**(23):3301-3307

[64] He N, Leng X, Zeng X. Systemic lupus erythematosus following human papillomavirus vaccination: A case-based review. International Journal of Rheumatic Diseases. 2022;**25**(10):1208-1212

[65] Grönlund O, Herweijer E, Sundström K, Arnheim-Dahlström L. Incidence of new-onset autoimmune disease in girls and women with pre-existing autoimmune disease after quadrivalent human papillomavirus vaccination: a cohort study. Journal of Internal Medicine. 2016;**280**(6):618-626

[66] Markowitz LE, Dunne EF, Saraiya M, Chesson HW, Curtis CR, Gee J, et al. Human papillomavirus vaccination: recommendations of the Advisory Committee on Immunization Practices (ACIP). MMWR - Recommendations and Reports. 2014;**63**(Rr-05):1-30

Chapter 4

Microvascular Involvement in Systemic Lupus Erythematosus Assessed by Nailfold Capillaroscopy: Correlations with Clinical and Biological Parameters

Alexandru Caraba, Deiana Roman, Stela Iurciuc,
Mihaela Nicolin and Mircea Iurciuc

Abstract

Systemic lupus erythematosus (SLE) is an autoimmune disease, mainly affecting women of childbearing age. Both macro- and microvascular involvements in SLE contribute to increased morbi-mortality associated with this disease. Microvascular involvement in SLE is found throughout the body. Multiple research methods linked to microvascular involvement were developed over time, nailfold capillaroscopy (NFC) being the most used both in the clinic and in research. In recent years, NFC has been used more and more in SLE patients. The aim of this chapter is to review the main capillaroscopic abnormalities that reflect the microvascular damage in SLE patients. Normal capillaries are significantly fewer than in healthy subjects, and capillaroscopic abnormalities are identified in almost 40–50% of SLE patients, consisting of tortuosity, hemorrhages, and modified morphology. On the other hand, the NFC score is higher than in healthy subjects. Some correlations are identified between capillaroscopic abnormalities and clinical and biological parameters. Disease activity is correlated with NFC score, and, on the other hand, with the abnormal capillaries morphology and hemmorhages. Raynaud's phenomenon is associated with dilated capillaries, while lupus nephritis with meandering capillaries. Further research is warranted in order to have a better understanding of microcirculation in SLE.

Keywords: microvascular involvement, nailfold capillaroscopy, systemic lupus erythematosus, capillaroscopic abnormalities, systemic lupus erythematosus complication

1. Introduction

Systemic lupus erythematosus (SLE) is a chronic autoimmune disease of unclear etiology, characterized by autoantibodies and immune circulation complexes

IntechOpen

production, generating the complement system activation, systemic inflammation, and protean clinical manifestations. Its symptoms can vary from mild to severe, potentially fatal manifestations [1]. This disease is considered as the prototype of autoimmune disease, which mainly affects the young women of childbearing years [2]. The pathogenesis of systemic lupus erythematosus (SLE) involves multiple humoral and cellular dysregulation [3]. Genetic susceptibility, environmental factors, or hormones lead to the appearance of the autoimmune response (preclinical period, characterized by the appearance of autoantibodies). Later, these autoantibodies and immune circulation complexes activated the complement system, generating inflammatory mediators and subsequent damage to different organs and systems (clinical period). SLE has an undulating evolution, with exacerbations and remissions. Over time, the accumulation of comorbidities related to irreversible destructive injuries is observed, due either to the disease itself or to the therapies used, generating high morbidity and mortality [4]. Antinuclear antibodies are the most characteristic of this disease, found in at least 95% of these patients [5].

The latest classification criterion for SLE was developed in 2019 by the European League Against Rheumatism (EULAR) in collaboration with the American College of Rheumatology (ACR). The aforementioned criterion must include at least one instance of antinuclear antibodies (ANA) being positive, representing a mandatory inclusion condition. Additionally, there are additive weighted criteria that have been separated into seven different groups, including clinical groups comprised of constitutional, hematologic, neuropsychiatric, mucocutaneous, serosal, musculoskeletal, and renal status, followed by three immunologic groups that include antiphospholipid antibodies, complement proteins, and SLE-specific antibodies. A total personal score of ten or above is indicative of the patient having a diagnosis of SLE [6].

2. Vascular involvement in SLE: micro- and macrovascular

Vascular involvement is considered the most serious feature of SLE, representing an important cause of morbidity and mortality in these patients. All types of blood vessels can be affected in the form of vasculopathy (non-inflammatory vascular lesions) or vasculitis (inflammatory vascular lesions with leukocytic infiltration and fibrinoid necrosis of the vascular walls). At the levels of large- and medium-sized arteries were described as atherosclerosis, thrombosis secondary to antiphospholipid syndrome, and vasculitis of visceral, coronary, and cerebral vessels. Microvascular involvement appeared in the form of cutaneous vasculitis, livedo reticularis, lupus nephritis, pulmonary and intestinal vasculitis, and pulmonary hypertension [7, 8].

3. Methods of microcirculation investigation in SLE patients

By using laser Doppler monitoring, color Doppler ultrasound, plethysmography, thermography, and nailfold capillaroscopy, microcirculation was assessed in SLE patients [3].

Nailfold capillaroscopy (NFC) is a noninvasive, repeatable method that is widely used in rheumatology, but not only [9]. Before the procedure, the patients were refrained from smoking and ingesting caffeine-containing drinks for at least 5 hours. The fingernail cuticles have not been removed for at least 1 month. The patients stayed for a minimum of 20 minutes in a room with a constant temperature of 22–25°C, with the hands positioned at the heart level. Nailfold capillaroscopy was performed on the second to fifth fingers, using a drop of immersion oil placed on the nailfold [10].

Standardization of nailfold capillaroscopic results distinguishes three patterns: normal pattern (hairpin shaped with a normal distribution) (**Figure 1**), non-specific pattern (tortuosity, crossing, meandering, and dilated capillaries) (**Figure 2**), scleroderma-like pattern (giant capillaries, microhemorrhages, avascularity, and neoangiogenesis) (**Figure 3**). Lower capillary density is defined by the reduction of capillary number below 7 capillaries per linear mm, counted at the distal row) [11].

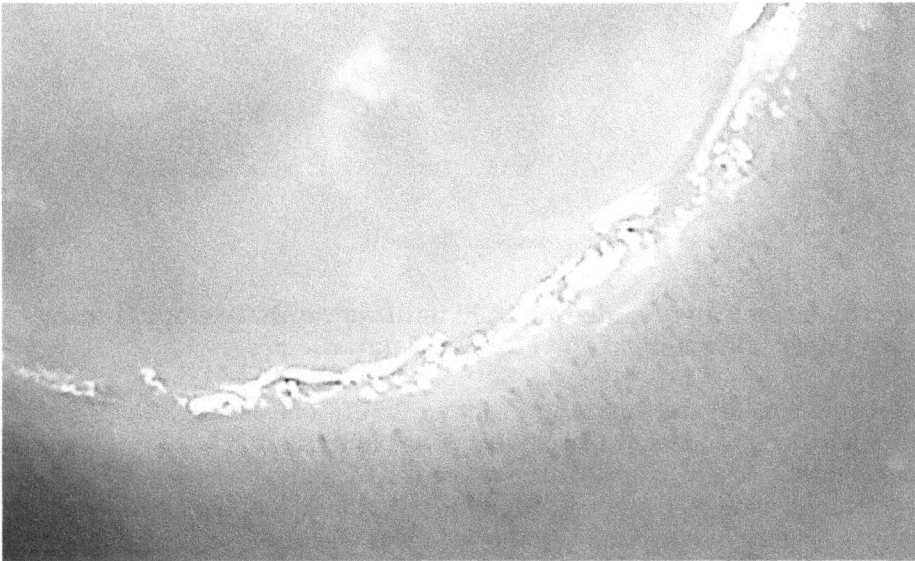

Figure 1.
NFC (×50): SLE: Normal pattern (personal collection).

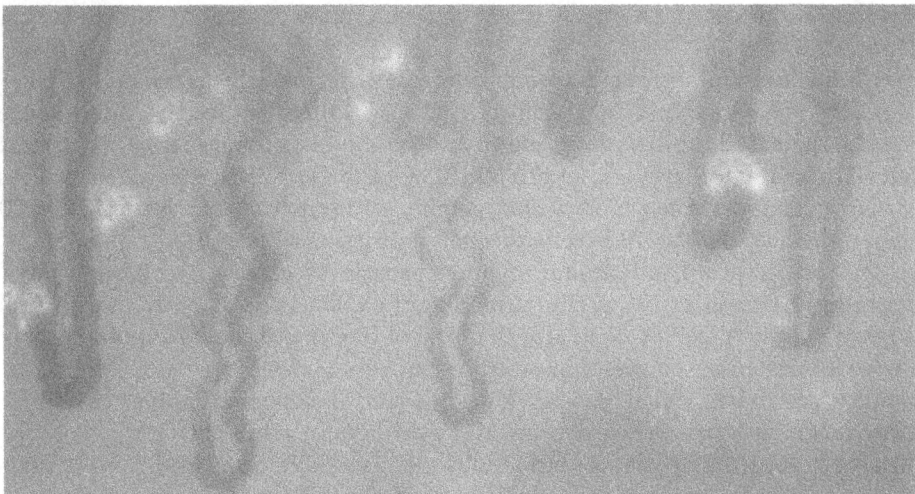

Figure 2.
NFC (×200): SLE: Non-specific pattern (personal collection).

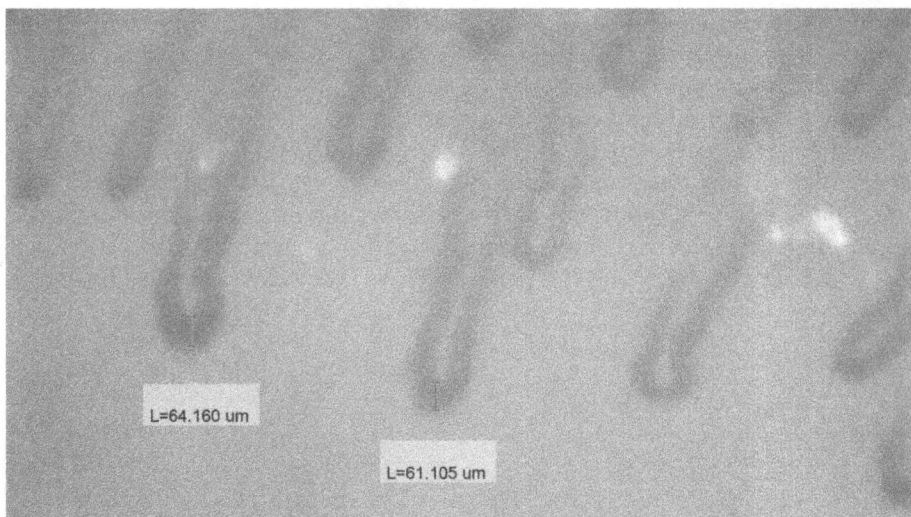

Figure 3.
NFC (×200): SLE: Scleroderma-like pattern (personal collection).

4. Microvascular involvement in SLE: nailfold capillaroscopy findings and correlation with clinical and biological parameters

SLE inflammatory mediators cause the damage of vascular endothelial cells, generating destruction and neovascularization. Over time, it was tried to find a unique model of microcirculation in SLE patients using NFC [12].

NFC findings are used for early diagnosis and prognosis of SLE. Until now, no unique model of nailfold capillaroscopic in SLE has been described. But Kabasakal et al. and Lambova and Muller-Ladner observed more frequent changes in SLE patients, such as tortuous capillaries and increased capillary diameter and length [13, 14]. Non-specific alterations were mainly described as capillaries with increased tortuosity and abnormal shapes, in addition to microhemorrhages [9]. A 'scleroderma-like' capillaroscopic pattern has been rarely observed (2–15%) in these patients [15, 16].

Five models of nailfold capillaroscopy were more frequently described in SLE patients. In 1986, Granier et al. described a pattern of tortuous and meandering capillaries with increased capillary loop length and prominent subpapillary plexus, exposing an increase in capillary loop length [17]. The probable SLE model was identified by McGill et al. as definite capillary enlargement without avascular areas [18]. In 2013, Lambova et al. defined an "SLE-type pattern" consisting of elongated capillaries, increased tortuosity, dilated capillaries, and a prominent subpapillary plexus [14]. The presence of capillary loops, the variability of capillary loop length, morphologic changes of venular plex visibility, and sludging of blood within said capillaries have also been identified by a number of other researchers as characteristic of SLE [19]. Subsequent, Bărbulescu et al. described a pattern with elongated capillaries with increased tortuosity, dilated capillaries, and a prominent subpapillary plexus [20].

In a study regarding patients with SLE by means of NFC 56, Shirani and Barahimi described an increased prevalence of the following capillaroscopic modifications: microvascular structure, decreased vascular density, enlarged capillary loops, microhemorrhages, as well as neoangiogenesis, amounting to 37.5, 78.6, 32.1, 16.1, and

25.0%, respectively. The authors identified a positive correlation between the duration of the disease and the presence of microhemorrhages (p = 0.043) [21].

The mean of capillaries density was significantly lower in SLE patients, compared to healthy controls [13, 14, 22], whereas in studies published by Caspary et al. [23], Studer et al. [24], Facina et al. [25], and Dancour et al. [26], no significant difference was found.

The capillary loop width was significantly higher in SLE patients compared to healthy controls in Ohtsuka study [27], whereas in two other studies, this difference was not significant [24, 28].

4.1 Cutaneous involvement in SLE

The skin is frequently affected in SLE, reaching up to 85–90%. Clinical manifestations include Raynaud's phenomenon, livedo reticularis, and cutaneous vasculitis [4].

The prevalence of Raynaud phenomenon (RP) in SLE is about 10–45%, having a more benign course, without tissue necrosis [14]. Endothelial dysfunction, abnormal adrenergic receptor reactivity, and inadequate release of neuropeptides or vasoactive mediators represent the main factors of RP. Due to its repetitive vasospasm, it leads to digital microinfarctions and ulcers or even gangrene of the distal portions of digits [29].

Secondary RP showed dilated and elongated capillaries, increased tortuosity, and prominent subpapillary plexus, but in some cases, the patients with secondary RP showed a scleroderma-like pattern [14].

Patients with SLE concomitantly presenting with RP have been found to be prone to the development of pulmonary arterial hypertension (PAH): by comparison, patients with SLE who did have PAH exhibited RP in 81% of the cases, while patients with SLE who did not associate PAH exhibited RP in only 56% of cases. After performing a univariate analysis, it was found that patients in which RP was present had a threefold increase in the risk of developing PAH. This finding supports the usage of this variable as a relevant indicator for the identification of this subpopulation of patients [16].

Caspary et al. performed a quantitative analysis of nailfold capillary morphology in 29 SLE patients with Raynaud phenomenon (RP), 29 RP-negative patients with SLE with the same duration of the disease, and 29 healthy controls. Tortuosity, meandering, and bushy capillaries were significantly increased in both groups of SLE patients without the influence of RP. Capillary density was lower, and the mean diameters of the capillary loops were higher in patients, especially when RP was present (p < 0.0005). SLE patients with the Raynaud phenomenon presented high capillary enlargement, correlated with the frequency of attacks [23].

In the study published by Zhao T et al. which was done on 85 SLE patients, RP was identified in 31.7% of patients. Nailfold capillaroscopy identified a normal pattern in 15.3% of patients, a non-specific pattern in 75.3% of patients, and scleroderma pattern in 9.4% of the studied lot. Capillaries dilatation was described in 81.5% of SLE patients with RP but only in 14% among the SLE patients without RP (p < 0.005) [12].

The most frequent NFC findings in the SLE and RP patients were enlarged capillaries and microhemorrhages [30]. In their study, Shenavandeh S and Habibi S. identified that minor NFC changes were present in 30.6% of patients and major changes in 63.9% of cases. Active skin involvement was associated with the disturbed distribution of capillaries (p < 0.004) [31].

Pavlov-Dolijanovic et al. studied 79 patients with SLE, of which 44 presented with RP, while 35 patients did not. The authors found significantly more frequent central nervous systemic involvement, as well as peripheral neuropathy, in patients with SLE and RP, while secondary Sjögren's syndrome was more common in patients with

SLE without RP. Nailfold capillaroscopy showed enlarged capillaries, avascular areas, capillary hemorrhages, and granular blood flow to be significantly more frequent in patients with SLE and RP compared to those without RP. A scleroderma-like pattern was more frequently identified in patients with RP [32].

Livedo reticularis is found in about 14–48% of SLE patients. It is produced by the dermal arterioles spasm and swelling of cutaneous venules [15].

Cutaneous vasculitis is observed in 19–28% of patients with SLE, being a leukocytoclastic vasculitis with immune complex deposition in the small vessels of the dermis and/or subcutaneous tissue [8].

All these patients presented NFC non-specific or scleroderma-like patterns [8].

4.2 Pulmonary involvement in SLE (interstitial lung disease; PAH)

In their study, Pallis et al. measured capillary density in 24 patients with systemic lupus erythematosus. The results of the study underlined the close correlation between nailfold capillary density and pulmonary gas transfer in patients with SLE. It was further hypothesized that nailfold capillary density might represent a feasible indicator of alveolar capillary density due to the fact that in patients with SLE, poor gas transfer may be dependent on alveolar capillary loss [22].

PAH, a potentially severe condition related to autoimmune rheumatic diseases, represents about 30% of all PAH cases in the adult population [33]. The prevalence of PAH associated with SLE patients varies from 0.5 to 14% according to the diagnosis methodology used [34, 35]. However, PAH development in SLE patients is associated with high morbidity and mortality [33, 36].

Development of PAH associated with SLE includes the following conditions: livedo reticularis, cutaneous vasculitis, Raynaud's phenomenon, serositis, and serologic abnormalities (anti-ribonucleoprotein, anti-cardiolipin antibodies, and high levels of serum endothelin-1 levels) [37, 38].

There is an increasing body of evidence linking NFC abnormalities with the presence and severity of PAH, underlining the role microcirculation might have in the development and pathogenesis of PAH [33, 39, 40].

In their study performed on 65 SLE patients (21 patients with SLE-PAH and 44 patients with SLE without PAH), Donnarumma et al. described the presence of scleroderma capillaroscopic pattern in 56.3% SLE-PAH versus 15.9% SLE without PAH patients (p = 0.002). Univariate analysis showed that the presence of Raynaud's phenomenon and scleroderma-like pattern were associated with PAH. On the other hand, by using multivariate analysis, the authors showed that a scleroderma capillaroscopic pattern was the sole variable associated with a significantly higher risk of PAH [33].

4.3 Lupus nephritis

In patients with lupus nephritis, Shenavandeh and Habibi did not identify any correlation between the capillary abnormalities and the presence of renal involvement (p > 0.05), except for the elongated capillary loops (p < 0.03) [31].

On the other hand, Ragab et al. identified a statistically significant positive correlation (p < 0.05) between the presence of meandering capillaries and 24 h urinary proteins. The explanation for this could be represented by the same vascular pathology affecting blood vessels in the kidney and nailfold region [41]. Kabasakal et al. showed that the renal vascular lesions are related to the SLE severity [13]. All studies showed that capillaroscopic abnormalities are present in LN. The existing differences in the reported results are due to the different selection of the studied SLE patients with LN, either based only on the renal histopathological examination or based on the urine and blood examinations.

4.4 Serology and SLE activity

NFC abnormalities have been detected in up to 36% of patients with SLE, with described correlations with autoantibodies anti-U1 ribonucleoprotein (U1RNP) [42].

In regards to autoantibody profiles and their correlation to the number of capillaries present in NFC, RNP positivity has been found to influence the severity of NFC findings in patients with SLE, showing a significant decrease in capillary numbers [14].

While significant differences were observed in regard to NFC patterns in patients with low disease activity when compared to those with high disease activity, the same did not apply to differences between anti-double stranded deoxyribonucleic acid, anti-Smith antibodies, and low complements [12]. The same results were reported by other studies. Kuryliszyn-Moskal A et al. evaluated the NFC changes in relation to the main serum endothelial cell activation markers and the disease activity of SLE in 80 patients. When NFC was performed, 33 patients with SLE showed a normal capillaroscopic pattern or mild changes (41.25%), while 47 patients with SLE presented moderate or severe abnormalities (58.75%). An NFC score of above 1 was more frequently associated with the presence of internal organ involvement. Between SLE patients with NFC score of above 1 and the control group, significant differences were found in the serum concentrations of endothelial cell activation markers. Moreover, a significant positive correlation was encountered between the severity of the NFC score and the Systemic Lupus Erythematosus Disease Activity Index (SLEDAI) [43]. Ciołkiewicz et al. identified a positive correlation between capillaroscopic score and disease activity (r = 0.339, p < 0.01) [44]. Kuryliszyn-Moskal et al. and Zhao et al. showed that the prevalence of microhemorrhage was higher in active SLE patients than in inactive cases [12, 45]. In their study, Shenavandeh and Habibi identified that minor NFC changes were present in 30.6% of patients and major changes in 63.9% of cases. Active SLE with higher activity was associated with severe NFC changes. Patients with active SLE have been found to have a higher incidence of microhemorrhages. In SLE patients with active skin involvement, the disturbed distribution pattern was more frequent, while subtle changes were less frequently observed compared to patients without active skin involvement [31].

Nasser et al. on 53 SLE patients, showed a significant correlation between NFC score and disease activity, expressed as SLEDAI (p = 0.021). The authors demonstrated that high levels of interferon I and interleukin 17A are found in active SLE. On the other hand, these mediators are involved in vascular injury, assessed by means of NFC [46].

It is known that SLE patients are prone to develop premature, accelerated, and extensive atherosclerosis. Farouk et al. showed that the lower density, longer, wider, and disorganized capillaries and tortuous and meandering capillaries were associated with the presence of atherosclerosis [47].

Data accumulated to date showed that there are statistically significant differences regarding the NFC abnormalities between SLE patients and healthy controls. SLE is an inflammatory autoimmune disease in which the mediators of autoimmunity and inflammation contribute to endothelial damage, with consequent vascular changes. Most studies have shown that the NFC scores correlate with the disease activity.

5. Conclusion

Data accumulated to date showed that there are statistically significant differences regarding the NFC abnormalities between SLE patients and healthy controls. SLE is an inflammatory autoimmune disease in which the mediators of autoimmunity and inflammation contribute to endothelial damage with consequent vascular changes. These vascular changes are highlighted by means of NFC. Indeed, there is no specific capillaroscopic pattern in SLE patients, but most studies have shown that the NFC scores correlate with the disease activity.

Studies on capillaroscopic aspects of SLE patients included a small number of people. Despite a small number of studied SLE patients, it was possible to conclude that the changed capillaroscopic pattern correlated with the presence of other vascular involvement at the level of different organs. Therefore, the presence of NFC changes in SLE patients requires the assessment of other organ damage in them (nephritis and pulmonary hypertension).

Due to the variable capillaroscopic repertoire found in SLE patients, multiple further multicenter studies are needed in order to clarify the NFC aspects and the correlation between them and clinical and laboratory parameters.

Acknowledgements

The present chapter has been published with the monetary support of the "Victor Babeş" University of Medicine and Pharmacy Timişoara.

Author details

Alexandru Caraba[1*], Deiana Roman[1], Stela Iurciuc[2], Mihaela Nicolin[3] and Mircea Iurciuc[2]

1 Department of 3rd Internal Medicine, Diabetes and Rheumatology, University of Medicine and Pharmacy "Victor Babeş" Timişoara, Romania

2 Department of Cardiology, University of Medicine and Pharmacy "Victor Babeş" Timişoara, Romania

3 Department of Cardiology, Military Hospital "Victor Popescu" Timişoara, Romania

*Address all correspondence to: alexcaraba@yahoo.com

IntechOpen

References

[1] Tsokos GC. Sytemic lupus erythematosus. The New England Journal of Medicine. 2011;**365**:2110-2121

[2] Jiménez S, Cervera R, Font J, Ingelmo M. The epidemiology of systemic lupus erythematosus. Clinical Reviews in Allergy and Immunology. 2003;**25**:3-12

[3] Fatemi A, Erlandsson BE, Emrani Z, et al. Nailfold microvascular changes in patients with systemic lupus erythematosus and their associative factors. Microvascular Research. 2019;**126**:103910

[4] Firestein GS, Budd RC, Gabriel SE, McInnes IB, O'Dell JR, Koretzky G, editors. Kelley & Firestein's Textbook of Rheumatology. 11th ed. Elsevier; 2020

[5] Arbuckle MR, McClain MT, Rubertone MV, et al. Development of autoantibodies before the clinical onset of systemic lupus erythematosus. The New England Journal of Medicine. 2003;**349**(16):1526-1533

[6] Aringer M, Costenbader K, Daikh D, et al. 2019 European league against rheumatism/American college of rheumatology classification criteria for systemic lupus erythematosus. Annals of the Rheumatic Diseases. 2019;**78**:1151-1159

[7] Kaul A, Gordon C, Crow MK, Touma Z, Urowitz MB, van Vollenhoven R, et al. Systemic lupus erythematosus. Nature Reviews. Disease Primers. 2016;**2**:16039

[8] Saygin D, Highland KB, Tonelli AR. Microvascular involvement in systemic sclerosis and systemic lupus erythematosus. Microcirculation. 2019;**26**(3):e12440

[9] Cutolo M, Melsens K, Wijnant S, et al. Nailfold capillaroscopy in systemic lupus erythematosus: A systematic review and critical appraisal. Autoimmunity Reviews. 2018;**17**:344-352

[10] Karbalaie A, Emrani Z, Fatemi A, et al. Practical issues in assessing nailfold capillaroscopic images: A summary. Clinical Rheumatology. 2019;**1**:12

[11] Smith V, Herrick AL, Ingegnoli F, et al. Standardisation of nailfold capillaroscopy for the assessment of patients with Raynaud's phenomenon and systemic sclerosis. Autoimmunity Reviews. 2020;**19**:102458

[12] Zhao T, Lin FA, Chen HP. Pattern of nailfold capillaroscopy in patients with systemic lupus erythematosus. Archives of Rheumatology. 2020;**35**(4):568-574

[13] Kabasakal Y, Elvins D, Ring E, McHugh N. Quantitative nailfold capillaroscopy findings in a population with connective tissue disease and in normal healthy controls. Annals of the Rheumatic Diseases. 1996;**55**:507-512

[14] Lambova SN, Muller-Ladner U. Capillaroscopic pattern in systemic lupus erythematosus and undifferentiated connective tissue disease: What we still have to learn? Rheumatology International. 2013;**33**:689-695

[15] Maricq HR, LeRoy EC, D'Angelo WA, et al. Diagnostic potential of *in vivo* capillary microscopy in scleroderma and related disorders. Arthritis and Rheumatism. 1980;**23**:183-188

[16] Furtado RN, Pucinelli ML, Cristo VV, et al. Scleroderma-like nailfold capillaroscopic abnormalities are associated with anti-U1-RNP antibodies

and Raynaud's phenomenon in SLE patients. Lupus. 2002;**11**:35-41

[17] Granier F, Vayssairat M, Priollet P, Housset E. Nailfold capillary microscopy in mixed connective tissue disease. Comparison with systemic sclerosis and systemic lupus erythematosus. Arthritis and Rheumatism. 1986;**29**:189-195

[18] McGill NW, Gow PJ. Nailfold capillaroscopy: A blinded study of its discriminatory value in scleroderma, systemic lupus erythematosus, and rheumatoid arthritis. Australian and New Zealand Journal of Medicine. 1986;**16**:457-460

[19] Wu P-C, Huang M-N, Kuo Y-M, et al. Clinical applicability of quantitative nailfold capillaroscopy in differential diagnosis of connective tissue diseases with Raynaud's phenomenon. Journal of the Formosan Medical Association. 2013;**112**:482-488

[20] Bărbulescu AL, Vreju AF, Buga AM, et al. Vascular endothelial growth factor in systemic lupus erythematosus - correlations with disease activity and nailfold capillaroscopy changes. Romanian Journal of Morphology and Embryology. 2015;**56**:1011-1016

[21] Shirani F, Barahimi L. Evaluation of the relationship between capillaroscopic symptoms and the severity of systemic lupus erythematous. Journal of Experimental Pathology. 2022;**3**(2):29-34

[22] Pallis M, Hopkinson N, Powell R. Nailfold capillary density as a possible indicator of pulmonary capillary loss in systemic lupus erythematosus but not in mixed connective tissue disease. The Journal of Rheumatology. 1991;**18**:1532-1536

[23] Caspary L, Schmees C, Schoetensack I, et al. Alterations of the nailfold capillary morphology associated with Raynaud phenomenon in patients with systemic lupus erythematosus. The Journal of Rheumatology. 1991;**18**(4):559-566

[24] Studer A, Hunziker T, Lütolf O, et al. Quantitative nailfold capillary microscopy in cutaneous and systemic lupus erythematosus and localized and systemic scleroderma. Journal of the American Academy of Dermatology. 1991;**24**(6):941-945

[25] Facina A, Pucinelli M, Vasconcellos M, et al. Capillaroscopy findings in lupus erythematosus. Clinical, Epidemiological, Laboratory and Therapeutic Investigation. 2006;**81**:523-528

[26] Dancour MA, Vaz JL, Bottino DA, Bouskela E. Nailfold videocapillaroscopy in patients with systemic lupus erythematosus. Rheumatology International. 2006;**26**(7):633-637

[27] Ohtsuka T. The relation between nailfold bleeding and capillary microscopic abnormality in patients with connective tissue diseases. International Journal of Dermatology. 1998;**37**(1):23-26

[28] Lefford F, Edwards JC. Nailfold capillary microscopy in connective tissue disease: A quantitative morphological analysis. Annals of the Rheumatic Diseases. 1986;**45**:741-749

[29] Sunderkötter C, Riemekasten G. Pathophysiology and clinical consequences of Raynaud's phenomenon related to systemic sclerosis. Rheumatology (Oxford). 2006;**45**(Suppl. 3):169-172

[30] Higuera V, Amezcua-Guerra LM, Montoya H, et al. Association of nail dystrophy with accrued damage and

capillaroscopic abnormalities in systemic lupus erythematosus. Journal of Clinical Rheumatology. 2016;**22**(1):13-18

[31] Shenavandeh S, Habibi S. Nailfold capillaroscopic changes in patients with systemic lupus erythematosus: Correlations with disease activity, skin manifestation and nephritis. Lupus. 2017;**26**(9):959-966

[32] Pavlov-Dolijanovic S, Damjanov NS, Vujasinovic Stupar NZ, et al. Is there a difference in systemic lupus erythematosus with and without Raynaud's phenomenon? Rheumatology International. 2013;**33**(4):859-865

[33] Donnarumma JFS, Ferreira EVM, Ota-Arakaki J, et al. Nailfold capillaroscopy as a risk factor for pulmonary arterial hypertension in systemic lupus erythematosus patients. Advances in Rheumatology. 2019;**59**:1

[34] Pope J. An update in pulmonary hypertension in systemic lupus erythematosus – do we need to know about it? Lupus. 2008;**17**:274-277

[35] Foïs E, Le Guern V, Dupuy A, et al. Noninvasive assessment of systolic pulmonary artery pressure in systemic lupus erythematosus: Retrospective analysis of 93 patients. Clinical and Experimental Rheumatology. 2010;**28**:836-841

[36] Qian J, Wang Y, Huang C, et al. Survival and prognostic factors of systemic lupus erythematosus-associated pulmonary arterial hypertension: A PRISMA-compliant systematic review and meta analysis. Autoimmunity Reviews. 2016;**15**:250-257

[37] Tselios K, Gladman DD, Urowitz MB. Systemic lupus erythematosus and pulmonary arterial hypertension: Links, risks, and management strategies. Open

access Rheumatology : Research and Reviews. 2016;**9**:1-9

[38] Huang C, Li M, Liu Y, et al. Baseline characteristics and risk factors of pulmonary arterial hypertension in systemic lupus erythematosus patients. Medicine (Baltimore). 2016;**95**(e2761):3

[39] Atsumi T, Bae S-C, Gu H, et al. Risk factors for pulmonary arterial hypertension in patients with systemic lupus erythematosus: A systematic review and expert consensus. ACR Open Rheumatology. 2023;**5**:663-676

[40] Wang D, Chen Z, Hou Z, et al. Characteristics and clinical significance of nailfold capillaroscopy in patients with systemic lupus erythematosus. Chinese Journal of Rheumatology. 2020;**12**:580-585

[41] Ragab O, Ashmawy A, Abdo M, Mokbel A. Nailfold capilloroscopy in systemic lupus erythematosus. The Egyptian Rheumatologist. 2011;**33**(1):61-67

[42] Ingegnoli F, Zeni S, Meani L, et al. Evaluation of nailfold videocapillaroscopic abnormalities in patients with systemic lupus erythematosus. Journal of Clinical Rheumatology. 2005;**11**:2958

[43] Kuryliszyn-Moskal A, Ciolkiewicz M, Klimiuk PA, Sierakowski S. Clinical significance of nailfold capillaroscopy in systemic lupus erythematosus: Correlation with endothelial cell activation markers and disease activity. Scandinavian Journal of Rheumatology. 2009;**38**(1):38-45

[44] Ciołkiewicz M, Kuryliszyn-Moskal A, Klimiuk PA. Analysis of correlations between selected endothelial cell activation markers, disease activity, and nailfold

capillaroscopy microvascular changes in systemic lupus erythematosus patients. Clinical Rheumatology. 2010;**29**(2):175-180

[45] Kuryliszyn-Moskal A, Klimiuk PA, Sierakowski S, Ciołkiewicz M. Vascular endothelial growth factor in systemic lupus erythematosus: Relationship to disease activity, systemic organ manifestation, and nailfold capillaroscopic abnormalities. Archivum Immunologiae et Therapiae Experimentalis. 2007;**55**:179-185

[46] Nasser M, Wadie M, Farid A, et al. Nailfold capillaroscopy in Egyptian systemic lupus erythematosus (SLE) patients: Correlation with demographic features and serum levels of IL 17A and IFNs I. Egyptian Rheumatology and Rehabilitation. 2023;**50**:47

[47] Farouk HM, Mohamed RM, Aboud FM, Hussein HT. Role of nail fold capillaroscopy as a method of early detection of atherosclerosis in systemic lupus erythematosus patients. QJM: An International Journal of Medicine. 2021;**114**(1):hcab100.071

Chapter 5

Sodium-Glucose Cotransporter 2 Inhibitors (SGLT-2i) in Lupus Nephritis

Abire Allaoui, Rita Aniq Filali, Amine Khalfaoui and Abdelhamid Naitlho

Abstract

Sodium-glucose cotransporter 2 inhibitors (SGLT-2i) have revolutionized the treatment of diabetic nephropathy. Their application was expanded to include other disorders, such as cardiovascular disease. Lupus nephritis is a significant complication of systemic lupus. Within the first 3 years of the disease, one-third of patients develop lupus nephritis. It is recognized as a leading cause of morbidity and mortality. Lupus nephritis therapy has improved with the use of corticosteroids, immunosuppressants such cyclophosphamide, mycophenolate mofetil, calcineurin inhibitors, and rituximab over the years. However, existing medications do not address all needs in the management of Lupus nephritis (LN) and are not always effective. According to new research, SGLT-2i may have potential for treating lupus nephritis due to their pleiotropic effects (anti-inflammatory, immunological, and hemodynamic implications). Recent trials using SGLT-2i in animals and humans have yielded encouraging outcomes in lupus nephritis. This review will explore the role of SGLT-2i in the management of lupus nephritis in addition to immunosuppressive medication.

Keywords: SGTL2 inhibitors, lupus, lupus nephritis, treatment, proteinuria

1. Introduction

Systemic lupus erythematosus (SLE) is a prototype of systemic autoimmune disease with alternating periods of remission and flares [1]. Approximately 33–50% of SLE patients develop organ involvement within 5 years of diagnosis [2]. The incidence and prevalence of SLE and LN differ based on the specific population under investigation and the diagnostic criteria employed to identify SLE and LN [2, 3]. Lupus nephritis (LN) is one of SLE's most common and severe complications [3]. Glomerulonephritis is the most prevalent type of LN. LN can progress to end-stage renal disease [3]. LN was linked to higher rates of illness and death, while SLE patients who did not develop LN had favorable overall outcomes in terms of survival [3]. Our understanding of the genetic and pathogenetic bases for LN has significantly advanced in recent decades [3, 4]. It is crucial to consider key risk factors to effectively assess and address progressive kidney disease. These include clinical parameters (proteinuria, glomerular filtration rate, complement levels, anti-dsDNA titer, and presence of antiphospholipid antibodies), kidney biopsy classification, and adherence to therapy [4].

Current treatments do not meet all needs in the management of LN and are not uniformly effective; they also carry significant risks and side effects, underscoring the need for novel therapeutic approaches [4]. While glucocorticoids and immunosuppressive agents such cyclophosphamide, mycophenolate mofetil, calcineurin inhibitors, and B-cell depletion therapy, remain the standard of care for LN, non-immunosuppressive therapies, such as renin-angiotensin-aldosterone system inhibitors, have always been part of the therapeutic arsenal of LN.

The concept of clinical response lacks unanimity, and there is an urgent need for uniform protocols to establish therapy response. A comprehensive response is typically achieved when the spot urinary protein-to-creatinine ratio is below 500 mg/g, the serum creatinine level reverts to the previous baseline or becomes normal, and there are less than five red blood cells per high-power field and no red blood cell casts in the urinary sediment. A partial response is achieved when the amount of protein in the urine decreases by more than 50% to a level that is below the threshold for kidney damage. This is indicated by a spot urinary protein-to-creatinine ratio of less than 3 g/g. Additionally, the serum creatinine level should be 15–25% higher or lower than the initial level. The number of red blood cells per high-power field should be less than 50% of the initial count, and there should be no red blood cell casts in the urine sediment [3]. Despite, all the advancements in the LN treatment, LN remains a substantial cause of morbidity and death among patients with SLE, and achieving clinical remission is not always possible.

Cardiovascular complications are also common and a leading cause of death in patients with SLE and LN. Patients with LN have multiple risk factors for cardiovascular complications, such as diabetes, dyslipidemia, and vascular inflammation [5].

Emerging evidence suggests that sodium-glucose cotransporter 2 inhibitors (SGLT-2i), a class of drugs primarily used to manage type 2 diabetes (T2D) and heart failure, may hold promise for treating lupus nephritis. These agents block reabsorption of glucose in the kidneys, leading to increased urinary glucose excretion and improved glycemic control [6]. Beyond their effects on blood sugar, SGLT2 inhibitors have demonstrated anti-inflammatory, antioxidant, and renoprotective properties that may be beneficial in autoimmune kidney diseases such as LN [7]. The unique renal and cardiac protective effects of SGLT2is in patients with chronic kidney disease (CKD) offer an attractive opportunity for SLE/LN management.

2. Sodium-glucose cotransporter 2

Sodium-glucose cotransporter 2 (SGTL2) belongs to a large family of membrane proteins located in the intestinal tract and proximal tubule, and is responsible for the transport of glucose, amino acids, vitamins, and some ions across the membrane of the epithelial intestine and proximal tubule in the kidneys. SGLT1 is predominantly found in the gastrointestinal tract, while SGLT2 is a renal protein, primarily expressed in the proximal tubule and accounts for 80–90% of glucose reabsorption, with the remaining 10–20% reabsorbed by SGLT1 [8]. SGLT-2 proteins have the physiological function of reabsorbing filtered glucose from the tubular lumen. Upon the discovery of the SGLT proteins, scientists found that phlorizin, an SGLT inhibitor, had been extensively researched for more than 150 years. However, it was only in recent decades that scientists uncovered its precise mechanism of action [7]. Phlorizin is derived from the root bark of the apple tree. In 1933, a limited number of individuals had a brief trial of the substance, during which scientists observed its ability to raise glucose levels in urine, decrease blood glucose levels, and inhibit the reabsorption of glucose. Its effect extended beyond the kidney. Due to its ability to impede glucose absorption in the intestine, limited oral absorption, and interference with glucose transport zones, it was considered inappropriate for human usage [7]. However, research on phlorizin played a crucial role in comprehending the functioning of sodium-glucose transporters, and scientists hypothesized that it might interfere with the activity of SGLTs. In 1995, researchers discovered that phlorizin effectively blocked the activity of both SGLT1 and SGLT2 [7]. Phlorizin's negative effects can be attributed to the presence of SGLT1 in several tissues and its crucial function in glucose absorption in the intestine. As scientists gained additional knowledge about phlorizin and SGLTs, they became intrigued by the potential of employing phlorizin as a basis for developing a diabetes treatment. Subsequent research efforts in the following decades were dedicated to enhancing the efficacy, selectivity, and duration of action of phlorizin derivatives targeted at SGLT2. This study led to the identification and evaluation of enhanced SGLT2 inhibitors [7].

Currently, four classes of SGLT-2i exist (canagliflozin, dapagliflozin, empagliflozin, and ertugliflozin), which reduce the reabsorption of filtered glucose, decrease the renal threshold for glucose, and promote urinary glucose excretion [9].

3. The revolution of SGLT-2i

Canagliflozin was the first SGLT-2 inhibitor approved on March 29, 2013, to be used in adult patients with type 2 diabetes to enhance blood glucose control in addition to diet and exercise [7]. These insulin-independent antihyperglycemic medications are now known to be pleiotropic agents with significant metabolic, cardiovascular, and renal benefits [9].

In addition to lowering glycated hemoglobin (HbA1c), fasting and postprandial plasma glucose levels, body weight, and blood pressure, SGLT2 inhibitors reduce the risk of a range of cardiovascular and renal outcomes, without increasing the risk of hypoglycemia [7].

Large clinical trials in patients with T2D with established cardiovascular disease or cardiovascular risk factors, heart failure, and CKD have shown that SGLT2 inhibitors confer cardiovascular and kidney protection [8]. In May of 2023, the FDA expanded the indication of dapagliflozin to include heart failure across the entire spectrum of left ventricular ejection fraction. This includes heart failure with mildly reduced ejection fraction (HFmrEF) and preserved ejection fraction (HFpEF) [8].

Four cardiovascular outcome trials showed that SGLT-2is has important effects on slowing the decline rate of the estimated glomerular filtration rate and decreasing albuminuria, in addition to a significant reduction in cardiovascular events. The nephroprotective efficacy of SGLT2is was extended to non-diabetic chronic kidney diseases such as IgA nephropathy [10]. Nephropathy reduces renal workload, thereby reducing intraglomerular pressure and regulating blood pressure [9, 10]. This has solved the management difficulties in patients with CKD and congestive heart failure [10].

SGLT2is are also used in Off-label indications such as the management of obesity in combination with glucagon-like peptide-1 receptor agonists and nonalcoholic fatty liver disease (NAFLD), as adjunctive therapy in patients with type 2 diabetes and NAFLD [7, 8].

In addition to its pleiotropic effects, SGLT-2is has been reported to be able to block lipopolysaccharide-induced and NOD-like receptor family pyrin domain containing 3 (NLRP3)-mediated inflammatory responses and regulate macrophage polarization via interplay with mammalian target of rapamycin (mTOR) and AMP-activated protein kinase pathways [10, 11]; hence, the promising effect of SGLT-2is to reducing inflammation, modulate endothelial dysfunction, and decelerate atherosclerosis, which are all impaired in the pathophysiology of SLE. Some recent studies with a small effective have found an antiproteinuric effect of empagliflozin in patients with LN [11].

4. Mechanistic effects of SGTL-2i

4.1 Renal effects

The effects of SGTL-2i on glomerular hemodynamic pathways have been analyzed in numerous studies, either in experimental models or in patients. SGLT2 inhibitors have demonstrated a reduction in hyperfiltration by inhibiting sodium reabsorption in the proximal tubule and have also shown an afferent renal arterial vasoconstriction and vasodilation of the renal efferent arteriole, similar to how angiotensin-converting enzyme inhibitors and angiotensin receptor blockers work [8], in addition to a decrease in intraglomerular pressure by restoring distal sodium delivery and therefore normalizing tubuloglomerular feedback [8, 12, 13].

Under hyperglycemic conditions, increased SGLT2 expression increases sodium and glucose reabsorption, which increases ATP-dependent tubular workload and oxygen consumption, both of which can result in hypoxia. As SGLT-2i reduces tubular workload, oxygen consumption, and hypoxia by reducing glucose and sodium reabsorption, they may also reduce the risk of acute kidney injury events and proximal biomarkers of acute kidney injury, such as kidney injury molecule-1 [8]. Interestingly, clinical studies have confirmed that EPO expression increases following SGLT2 inhibition [14, 15]. Therefore, it was not surprising to see that the risk of anemia, which was an independent predictor of renal and cardiovascular outcomes, and the start of anemia treatment were significantly reduced with canagliflozin in a sizable multi-national kidney outcome trial [16].

4.2 Effects on blood pressure

The systolic and diastolic blood pressures were reduced by approximately 4 and 2 mmHg, respectively, by SGLT-2i. It is likely that SGLT-2i lowers blood pressure through different contributing variables [8]. Increased natriuresis and osmotic diuresis in conjunction with decreases in extracellular volume and plasma volume are believed to be responsible for SGLT-2i's ability to control blood pressure, and according to human clinical trials, SGLT-2i has a positive impact on blood pressure variability, endothelial function, and arterial stiffness [8, 13, 17]. These results suggest that sympathoinhibition may be a modulator of the beneficial effects of SGLT-2i on the kidneys and perhaps the cardiovascular system [8].

4.3 Effects in non-diabetic patients

In patients with CKD, the DAPA-CKD trial demonstrated a decreased risk of kidney failure, hospitalization for heart failure or death from cardiovascular causes, and all-cause mortality, with statistically significant effects in reducing the risk of kidney failure both in the subgroup of patients with and without type 2 diabetes [17].

Furthermore, the EMPEROR-Reduced and DAPA-HF trials showed that SGLT-2i lowered the risk of heart failure hospitalizations or cardiovascular death and slowed the progression of kidney function decline in patients with heart failure. They reduced the ejection fraction, both with and without type 2 diabetes [18, 19]. These three clinical trials showed that SGLT-2i has positive effects in patients with type 2 diabetes. If used in clinical practice, it can revolutionize the management of a wide spectrum of high-risk CKD patients [8].

4.4 Immunological effects

Unexpectedly, SGLT2i therapy also has immunological effects that go beyond metabolic effects. Through the induction of regulatory T-cell production, they have a significant effect on the development of germinal centers and creation of autoreactive plasma cells in the spleen [17].

It appears that SGLT-2i inhibits both podocyte and macrophage mTOR activation [18, 19]. The significance of mTOR blocking in patients with SLE is highlighted by the well-established roles that mTOR plays in proinflammatory lineage formation [20], podocyte and endothelial cell dysfunction [21], and adaptive immune system activation [22]. In addition to their protective effects on the kidneys and heart, SGLT-2i may function as an adjuvant immunomodulatory therapy for SLE, partly through mTOR inhibition [10].

Higher ketone body concentrations decrease monocyte production of interleukin-1b and inhibit the Nod-like receptor pyrin domain-containing protein 3 (NLRP3) inflammasome [23, 24]. These inflammatory mediators are significant inflammatory pathways that may have a major impact on the onset and course of renal disease [25]. Some clinical trials with SGLT-2i in patients with type 2 diabetes have revealed important effects on inflammatory mediators, including decreases in urine IL-6 and MCP-1, as well as serum tumor necrosis factor receptor 1 and IL-6 [8, 17].

Finally, SGLT2is can inhibit apoptosis and the production of reactive oxygen species and attenuates glomerular atrophy, kidney fibrosis, and kidney dysfunction [18, 19].

5. Proof of concept

A study conducted in 2023 confirmed the renoprotective effect of SGLT2 inhibitors in lupus mice, underscoring the role of non-immunosuppressive treatment in improving renal function in classic autoimmune kidney diseases, such as LN [20]. The levels of mouse anti-dsDNA IgG-specific antibodies, serum creatinine, and proteinuria markedly decreased. From a histological perspective, glomerular and tubulointerstitial damage was reduced by empagliflozin administration [20].

An observational international cohort study found that the use of SGLT2i in the management of glomerular/systemic autoimmune diseases with proteinuria was associated with a significant reduction in proteinuria, irrespective of the underlying disease [21]. An SGLT2i (empagliflozin) add-on to sustained immunosuppressive treatment showed a promising reduction in proteinuria (~50% reduction within 8 weeks) in a small case series of five active individuals with LN [10].

Another small study (n = 9) showed significantly reduced proteinuria in patients with lupus nephritis [20].

In a recent cohort study of a total of 31,790 patients, the propensity matched 1775 matched pairs of SGLT2i users and nonusers (N = 3550), the patients had a mean age of 57 years, with 85% of them being women. This study showed that SGLT2i use was associated with a significantly lower risk of incident lupus nephritis (AHR, 0.55; 95% CI, 0.40–0.77), dialysis (AHR, 0.55; 95% CI, 0.40–0.77), kidney transplant (AHR, 0.14; 95% CI, 0.03–0.62), heart failure (AHR, 0.65; 95% CI, 0.53–0.78), and all-cause mortality (AHR, 0.35; 95% CI, 0.26–0.47) than SGLT2i non-use in patients with SLE and type 2 diabetes [22]. Since individuals with systemic lupus face a greater risk of developing cardiovascular illness as a result of systemic inflammation, it seems that SGLT2i could potentially provide the additional advantage of decreasing the risk of heart failure in this particular group of patients [22]. The use of SGLT2 inhibitors in systemic lupus erythematosus provides both kidney-protective and heart-protective advantages.

Considering this evidence, SGLT2i have been recommended as a treatment adjuvant for LN in the recent KDIGO recommendations for LN management published in 2024 [23].

6. Overrated expectations?

In a trial, 38 patients with LN were treated with dapagliflozin add-on therapy, and the safety profile as a primary endpoint was acceptable; however, the secondary endpoints revealed no improvement in SLE Disease Activity Index scores or proteinuria (among 17 patients with LN) [10]. The authors proposed two major explanations. First, <50% of the patients with LN were on renin-angiotensin-aldosterone system inhibitors, which has been postulated to be required for SGLT2is to enhance their action. Another possible reason might be attributed to the fact that the participants had a relatively long LN duration and were resistant to several immunosuppressants in the past [10].

7. Concerns of using SGTL2i in LN

7.1 Increased risk for infections in lupus

Urinary tract infections are a typical side effect of SGLT2is because they increase glucose availability in the urinary tract [22]. Urinary tract infections are a concern for SLE patients because they are prone to various infections. Nonetheless, only one patient (2.63%) experienced urinary tract infections in a trial, which was not higher than that in non-SLE large-scale clinical trials [10].

As SGLT-2 inhibitors also increase the risk of genital mycotic infections, both male and female patients with a history of these illnesses should be closely monitored [23].

Therefore, patients undergoing SGLT-2i therapy should be closely monitored for clinical features of urinary tract infections, such as dysuria, urinary frequency, urgency, and suprapubic discomfort. If present, urinalysis should be performed to rule out infections [24].

7.2 Vascular problems

Before initiating canagliflozin and ertugliflozin, patients should be screened for risk factors for lower limb amputations, such as peripheral vascular disease, history of amputations, and neuropathy, especially in patients with SLE, and should be routinely monitored for infections or ulcer formations of the lower extremities, as non-traumatic lower limb amputations have been reported [25].

7.3 Osteoporosis

SGLT2 inhibitors are associated with increased incidence of bone fractures. Increased fracture risk has been observed with canagliflozin, occurring 12 weeks after treatment initiation [26]. Potential mechanisms for fracture include volume contraction leading to dizziness and falls, and possible effects on calcium, phosphate, and vitamin D homeostasis, leading to a reduction in bone mineral density [27]. This risk can increase in patients with SLE treated with corticosteroids.

8. Conclusion

Currently, there is little data supporting the use of iSGLT-2 in lupus nephritis; the studies were small observational series and case studies with positive effects on renal and cardiovascular protection. Further randomized experiments are required to confirm these encouraging results. On SGTL-2i, this specific patient group should be regularly monitored for osteoporosis and the risk of genital and urinary infections.

Acknowledgements

All authors acknowledge Dr. Amine Azzaz for his assistance in providing us with articles published about sodium-glucose cotransporter 2 inhibitors (SGLT-2i) in Lupus nephritis.

Conflict of interest

The authors declare no conflict of interest.

Notes/thanks/other declarations

No declarations.

Author details

Abire Allaoui[1,2,3*], Rita Aniq Filali[1], Amine Khalfaoui[4] and Abdelhamid Naitlho[1]

1 Internal Medicine Department, Mohammed VI University of Health and Sciences, Casablanca, Morocco

2 Clinical Immunology, Autoimmunity and Inflammation Laboratory (LICIA), Faculty of Medicine and Pharmacy, Hassan II University, Casablanca, Morocco

3 Mohammed VI Center of Research and Innovation, Rabat, Morocco

4 Nephrology Department, Mohammed VI University of Health and Sciences, Casablanca, Morocco

*Address all correspondence to: abire.allaoui@gmail.com

IntechOpen

References

[1] Manson JJ, Rahman A. Systemic lupus erythematosus. Orphanet Journal of Rare Diseases. 2006;**1**:6

[2] Bell CF, Ajmera MR, Meyers J. Evaluation of costs associated with overall organ damage in patients with systemic lupus erythematosus in the United States. Lupus. 2022;**31**(2):20211

[3] Anders HJ, Saxena R, Zhao MH, Parodis I, Salmon JE, Mohan C. Lupus nephritis. Nature Reviews Disease Primers. 2020;**6**(1):7

[4] Avasare R, Drexler Y, Caster DJ, et al. Management of lupus nephritis: New treatments and updated guidelines. Kidney360. 2023;**4**(10):150311

[5] Katayama Y, Yanai R, Itaya T, Nagamine Y, Tanigawa K, al. Risk factors for cardiovascular diseases in patients with systemic lupus erythematosus: An umbrella review. Clinical Rheumatology. 2023;**42**(11):293141

[6] Perkovic V, Jardine MJ, Neal B, Bompoint S, Heerspink HJL, Charytan DM, et al. Canagliflozin and renal outcomes in type 2 diabetes mellitus and nephropathy. The New England Journal of Medicine. 2019;**380**(24):2295306

[7] Nelinson DS, Sosa JM, Chilton RJ. SGLT2 inhibitors: A narrative review of their efficacy and safety. Journal of Osteopathic Medicine. 2021;**121**(2):22939

[8] Sen T, Heerspink HJL. A kidney perspective on the mechanism of action of sodium glucose co-transporter 2 inhibitors. Cell Metabolism. 2021;**33**(4):732-739. DOI: 10.1016/j.cmet.2021.02.016

[9] PLOSKER, Greg L. Canagliflozin: A review of its use in patients with type 2 diabetes mellitus. Drugs. 2014;**74**:807-824

[10] Wang H, Li T, Sun F, Liu Z, Zhang D, Teng X, et al. Safety and efficacy of the SGLT2 inhibitor dapagliflozin in patients with systemic lupus erythematosus: A phase I/II trial. RMD Open. 2022;**8**(2):e002686

[11] Morales E, Galindo M. SGLT2 inhibitors in lupus nephropathy, a new therapeutic strategy for nephroprotection. Annals of the Rheumatic Diseases. 2022;**81**(9):13378

[12] Kidokoro K, Cherney DZI, Bozovic A, Nagasu H, Satoh M, Kanda E, et al. Evaluation of glomerular hemodynamic function induced by empagliflozin in diabetic mice using in vivo imaging. Circulation. 2019;**140**(4):30315

[13] Cherney DZI, Perkins BA, Soleymanlou N, Maione M, Lai V, Lee A, et al. Renal hemodynamic effects of sodium-glucose cotransporter 2 inhibition in patients with type 1 diabetes mellitus. Circulation. 2014;**129**(5):58797

[14] Lambers Heerspink HJ, de Zeeuw D, Wie L, Leslie B, List J. Dapagliflozin a glucose-regulating drug with diuretic properties in subjects with type 2-diabetes. Diabetes, Obesity & Metabolism. 2013;**15**(9):85362

[15] Mazer CD, Arnaout A, Connelly KA, Gilbert JD, Glazer SA, Verma S, et al. Sodium-glucose cotransporter 2 inhibitors and type 2 diabetes: Clinical pearls for in-hospital initiation, in-hospital management, and post-discharge. Current Opinion in Cardiology. 2020;**35**(2):17886

[16] Oshima M, Neuen BL, Jardine MJ, Bakris G, Edwards R, Levin A, et al. Effects of canagliflozin on anemia in patients with type 2 diabetes and chronic kidney disease: A post-hoc analysis from the CREDENCE trial. The Lancet Diabetes and Endocrinology. 2020;**8**(11):90314

[17] Dekkers CCJ, Gansevoort RT. Sodium-glucose cotransporter 2 inhibitors: Extending the indications to non-diabetic kidney disease? Nephrology Dialysis Transplantation. 2020;**35** (Suppl. 1):i3342

[18] Verma S, Jüni P, Mazer CD. Pumps, pipes, and filters: Do SGLT2 inhibitors cover it all? The Lancet. 2019;**393**(10166):35

[19] Chang WT, Wu CC, Liao IC, et al. Dapagliflozin protects against doxorubicin-induced nephrotoxicity associated with nitric oxide pathway-A translational study. Free Radical Biology and Medicine. 2023;**208**:103-111. DOI: 10.1016/j.freeradbiomed.2023.08.013

[20] Zhao XY, Li SS, He YX, Yan LJ, Lv F, Liang QM, et al. SGLT2 inhibitors alleviate podocyte damage in lupus nephritis by decreasing inflammation and enhancing autophagy. Annals of the Rheumatic Diseases. 2023;**82**(10):132840

[21] Caravaca-Fontán F, Stevens K, Padrón M, Huerta A, Montomoli M, Villa J, et al. Inhibition of sodium-glucose cotransporter 2 in primary and secondary glomerulonephritis. Nephrology Dialysis Transplantation. 2024;**39**(2):32840

[22] Yen FS, Wang SI, Hsu CC, Hwu CM, Wei JC. Sodium-glucose cotransporter-2 inhibitors and nephritis among patients with systemic lupus erythematosus. JAMA Network Open. 2024;7(6):e2416578. DOI: 10.1001/jamanetworkopen.2024.16578

[23] Rovin BH, Ayoub IM, Chan TM, Liu ZH, Mejía-Vilet JM, Floege J. KDIGO 2024 clinical practice guideline for the management of LUPUS NEPHRITIS. Kidney International. 2024;**105**(1):S169

[24] Hall V, Kwong J, Johnson D, Ekinci EI. Caution advised with dapagliflozin in the setting of male urinary tract outlet obstruction. BML Case Reports. 2017;**2017**:bcr2017219335

[25] Scheen AJ. An update on the safety of SGLT2 inhibitors. Expert Opinion on Drug Safety. 2019;**18**(4):295311

[26] Watts NB, Bilezikian JP, Usiskin K, et al. effects of canagliflozin on fracture risk in patients with type 2 diabetes mellitus. The Journal of Clinical Endocrinology and Metabolism. 2016;**101**(1):157-166. DOI: 10.1210/jc.2015-3167

[27] Fralick M, Kim SC, Schneeweiss S, Kim D, Redelmeier DA, Patorno E. Fracture risk after initiation of use of canagliflozin: A cohort study. Annals of Internal Medicine. 2019;**170**(3):15563

Chapter 6

Placental Malperfusion in Maternal Diseases

Rosete Nogueira and Filipe Soares Nogueira

Abstract

Pregnancy loss occurs throughout gestation and can be divided into specific mechanisms, the frequency of which varies by trimester. Placental pathologies are associated with obstetric syndromes or scenarios across the second and third trimester resulting from multiple maternal diseases often related to poor placental perfusion. Chronic placental hypoxia based on mechanism could be preuterine (related to hypoxemia), uterine (due to injury of the uterine vessels), and postuterine (due to fetoplacentar vascular compromise). Complex vascular fetomaternal processes result in common and combined placentar pathological features that are timing-dependent. Immediate life-saving procedures or long-term care related, among others, to hypoxic encephalopathy can be improved by anticipating preventive measures that encompass the currently designated adult-onset diseases of placental origin.

Keywords: placental malperfusion, hypertensive disorders in pregnancy, lupus erythematosus, lupus anticoagulant, antiphospholipid antibodies, thrombophilia, diabetes mellitus, gestational diabetes

1. Introduction and general consideration

Placental pathologies are associated with obstetric syndromes or scenarios related to multiple maternal diseases, frequently resulting in placental abnormalities, malperfusion, and loss of functional capacity [1–3].

Tightly controlled interactions between the immune, endocrine, and metabolic systems during pregnancy are necessary in order to establish proper placentation, nurture, and immune homeostasis [4]. Disbalance in these interactions is considered to be a base of many pregnancy-associated disorders including hypertensive disorders namely preeclampsia and HELLP (Hemolysis, Elevated Liver enzymes, Low Platelet) syndrome [4].

Placental pathologies are often combined into multiple and complex lesions, resulting in different maternal-fetal morbidity and mortality associated across complex timing-dependent processes linked to immediate procedures or long-term care related to others with hypoxic encephalopathy [3]. Successful pregnancies require an even balance of coagulation and fibrinolysis in order to secure stabilization of the basal plate as well as adequate placental perfusion.

The development of thrombotic disorders is a major threat to young women during pregnancy. It is one of the main causes of pregnancy-related disorders, which may also result in harm to the conceptus.

Preventive measures for what is currently designated as adult-onset diseases of placental origin must be part of clinical guidance standards in primary health care [4]. Although not covered in their entirety in this chapter, serve to alert us to their relationship with childhood and adult diseases and consequently make us reflect on ways of preventing them.

Therefore, promoting studies that anticipate the assessment of the functional capacity of the placenta in real-time, similar to what happens with fetal assessment, is essential to prevent the critical reduction of the placental exchange membrane. Despite the limitations of the fetal:placental weight ratio, recent studies approach placental volume may be more promising in evaluating placental function/dysfunction [1–6].

2. Hypertensive disorders in pregnancy

2.1 Gestational and chronic hypertension and preeclampsia

2.1.1 Definition

Hypertensive disorder in pregnancy is defined as a blood pressure of 140/90 or more over two readings at least 4 hours apart and is categorized as pre-pregnancy hypertension or chronic hypertension; gestational hypertension or new-onset hypertension during pregnancy without features of preeclampsia; preeclampsia/eclampsia defined as new-onset hypertension during pregnancy with proteinuria or other specified clinical features; HELLP syndrome (Hemolytic anemia, Elevated Liver enzymes, Low Platelet) is considered a preeclampsia with severe features [4, 6, 7]. Chronic hypertension may be associated with superimposed preeclampsia, and this is often further classified as early or late onset with the dividing gestational age (GA) being 34 weeks, the first being associated with a poorer prognosis [8].

2.1.2 Demography

Chronic hypertension is rising in prevalence due to an increase in maternal age during pregnancy and the obesity epidemic. Hypertension during pregnancy (gestational hypertension) is common, occurring in approximately 10% of pregnancy [9], and chronic hypertension complicates about 5% of pregnancies [7, 9, 10] and is higher in multiparous and in previous pregnancies complicated by preeclampsia [7]. The rate of preeclampsia is reported at about 2 to 7%, being higher between Hispanic and African-American women [11]. The prevalence of gestational hypertension ranges from 6 to 17% [7]. HELLP syndrome incidence varies from 0,5 to 7,6 per 1000 deliveries and between 8 and 24% of cases with severe preeclampsia/eclampsia [7]. HELLP syndrome occurs in a circulatory inflammatory milieu that might in turn participate in a complex interplay involving an innate and adaptive immune understudied field [4]. A disbalanced response may lead to prolonged immunoactivation and tissue damage that implies a risk of serious morbidity and mortality to both the mother and the fetus during pregnancy [4, 7].

2.1.3 Etiology

Hypertension causes vary and differ according to specific hypertensive diagnoses. Chronic hypertension is associated with genetic and epigenetic factors, race, age, body mass index (BMI), dietary factors, and adrenergic tónus. Gestational hypertension and preeclampsia share many risk factors and epidemiologic associations. However, there are some significant differences in their biomarker profiles, risk factors, and outcomes that suggest they may relate to distinct pathogens [12, 13]. Although many aspects of pathophysiology related to the valency of vascular conversion have been well-described, namely in preeclampsia, the specific etiology remains elusive. Due to the abnormal vascular adaptations, placental hypoxia, chronic ischemia-reperfusion injury, and increased oxidative stress develop [14–16]. Placental hypoxia leads to the release of bioactive and vasoactive factors into the maternal circulation as a truncated form of the vascular endothelial growth factor (VEGF) receptor that retains the ligand binding such as soluble Fms-like tyrosine kinase (sFLT-1) and soluble endoglin (sENG) acting as antiangiogenic factors bind to neutralize and decrease circulating concentrations of the proangiogenic factors (VEGF) and placental growth factor (PIGF), leading to generalized endothelial damage and antiangiogenic state (characteristic of preeclampsia). Also, immune dysregulation or maladaptation and abnormal proinflammatory states in early placentogenesis have been suggested to be a causative feature leading to secondary trophoblast dysfunction [4, 16], justifying the same HELLP occurrence [4]. Other factors involved are related to nulliparity, changes of paternity, long interpregnancy intervals, and ova and sperm donor-conceived pregnancies [17, 18].

2.1.4 Risk factors

Maternal factors playing an increased risk of pregnancy hypertensive disorders are antiphospholipid antibody syndrome; previous preeclampsia (increasing the risk of recurrence in parallel with the severity of the previous manifestation); chronic hypertension; pregestational diabetes; woman born small for gestational age; history of any form of hypertension previous pregnancies; and certain complications in previous pregnancies (e.g., fetal growth restriction (FGR), abruption, and stillbirth) are more likely to have circulatory disorders namely preeclampsia [19]. Paternal factors play a role as well, with men who have fathered a preeclampsia pregnancy more likely to father another pregnancy complicated with precalmpsia with the same or new partner. Also, placental features impose an increased risk of hypertension in pregnancy, like hydrops (especially trisomy 13 and triploidy), molar gestations, and multiple gestations, and are higher with higher order multiple births [19]. Other risk factors include unexplained FGR, urinary tract, and periodontal infections [19].

2.1.5 Pathology

2.1.5.1 Gross placental findings

Placentas complicated with maternal hypertensive disorders share gross pathologic features that correlate with the chronicity and severity of the hypertension. Maternal vascular malperfusion (MVM) complicate placentas are often small for gestational age by weight (less than 10th percentile). The umbilical cord may be thin (less than 0,8 cm at term) [1, 2]. Other commonly present features include infarcts (hypertensive-type) and features of chronic or acute abruption (infarction hematomas/rounded intraplacental hematomas with (or not) detachment of the placenta from its decidual seat) [1, 2]. Increased perivillous/intervillous fibrin may be grossly identified but not to the point of massive perivillous fibrin deposition/maternal floor infarct [1, 2]. Increased villous stromal or intervillous calcifications are often associated with other features of MVM [1, 2]. The HELLP syndrome can share some pathophysiological traits with preeclampsia (attributed to deficient spiral artery remodeling and shallow trophoblast invasion) [20]. Early onset hypertensive placentas are more likely to show hypoplasia with placental weights less than 10th percentile, thin umbilical cords [20]. Curiously, some authors found that HELLP syndrome placentas were heavier and had fewer infarcts and retroplacental hematomas (RPH) than preeclampsia [20]. Abruption is more related to preeclampsia, and pathologically, this results in an RPH (**Figure 1**).

2.1.5.2 Microscopic findings

The most characteristic microscopic MVM associate lesions are distal villous hypoplasia or accelerated villous maturation [1, 2] infarcts, usual and hypertensive type, infarction hematoma/rounded intraplacental hematoma [1, 2] distal villous

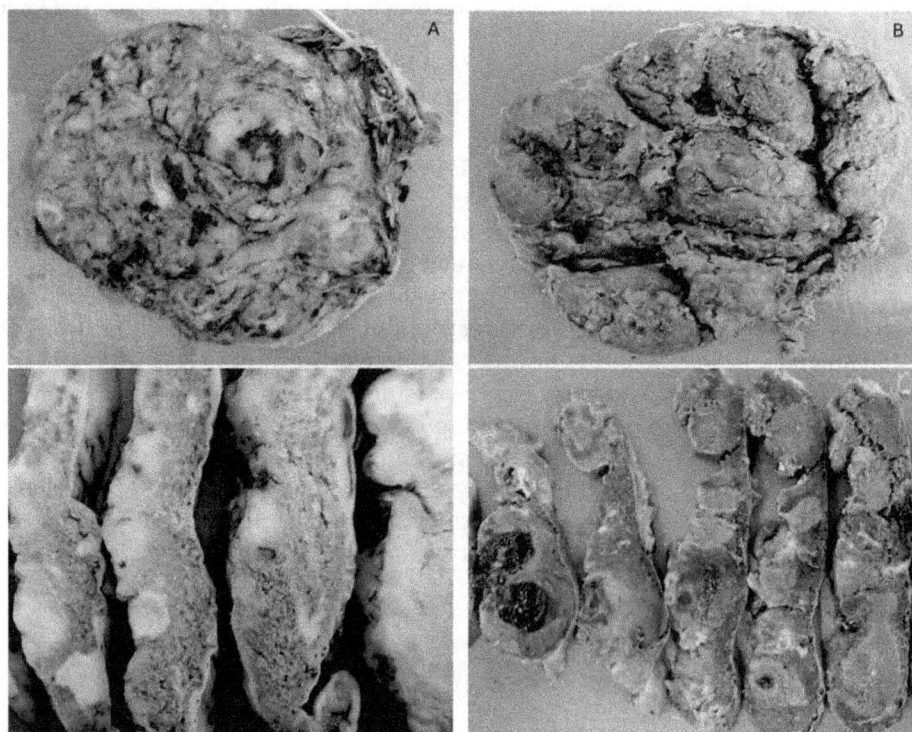

Figure 1.
Placenta with multiple gross features of maternal vascular malperfusion (MVM). (A), increased fibrin / fibrinoid in basal plate (top) and multiple old infarcts (bottom) in the cut section of the placenta from a woman with chronic hypertension. (B), maternal surface without sigificative lesions (top) and several intramural hematomas more seen in the cut section of a placenta from a woman with severe preeclampsia.

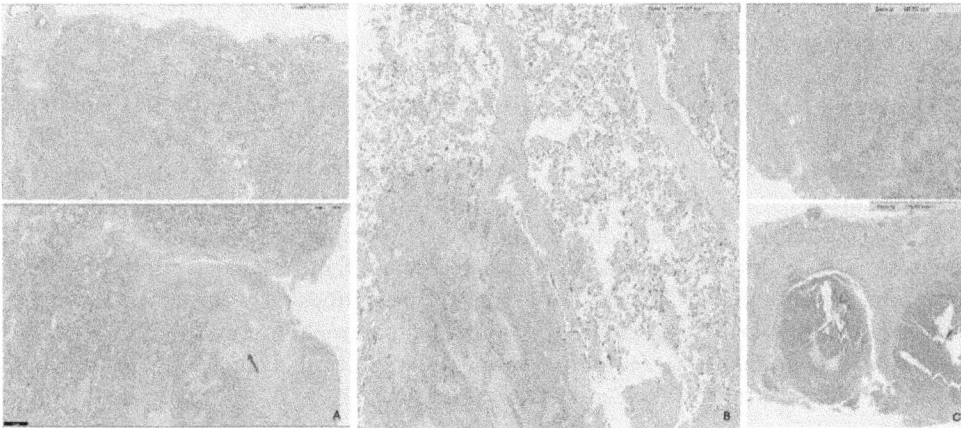

Figure 2.
Placental several microscopic features of maternal vascular malperfusion (MVM). (A), Intermediate-age hypertensive infarct with colapse villi and loss of the intervillous space (top), increased basal and perivillous fibrin associated with a palcental infarct (bottom) and decidual vasculopathy (arrow) from a woman with chronic hypertension. (B), low-power view of 32-week preeclamptic placenta with accelerated villous maturation, increase syncytial knots, hypertensive type infarct and distal villous hypoplasia. (C), old-age infarct usual type, (top) and fresh abruptio with early infarction of villous tissue, the clot below is elevating the decidua basalis (bottom), from a woman with severe preeclampsia.

hypoplasia (DVH) and/or accelerated villous maturation (AVM), abruption, intra-villous hemorrhage, RPH with associated infarct, decidual hemorrhage, placental parenchymal compression; increased perivillous fibrin; decidual arteriopathy with or without acute atherosis, thrombus, untransformed decidual (basal plate) vessels; increased trophoblast fibrinoid islands; villous agglutination; increased syncytial trophoblastic knots; trophoblastic giant cells in the decidual basal, decidual laminar necrosis, diffuse decidual leukocytoclastic necrosis (**Figure 2**).

The diagnosis of these disorders including placental hypertension cannot be based on the placental findings alone, and clinical correlation is necessary because some fetal growth restriction placentas without clinical hypertension have features of MVM including decidual arteriopathy.

3. Lupus erythematosus

3.1 Definition

Lupus erythematosus (LE) is a chronic autoimmune disease, characterized by widespread inflammation with tissue damage across various organs systems [21]. During pregnancy, women often experience flares or exacerbation of symptoms, which may lead to several maternal and fetal health complications. The most common form is systemic lupus erythematosus (SLE), which affects multiple organ systems.

3.2 Demography

Lupus affects people of all ages, but it is most diagnosed in women of childbearing age, particularly between 15 and 55 years old [22]. Women are affected approximately nine times more often than men. The prevalence of lupus varies by ethnicity; it is more common in people of African, Hispanic, Asian, and Native American descent than in Caucasians [23].

3.3 Etiology

The exact cause of LE is unknown, but it is believed to be a disease that results of a combination of genetic, hormonal, environmental, and immunological factors. Some specific etiological factors include a family history of lupus or other autoimmune diseases that can increase the risk; exposure to certain factors such as sunlight, infections, and certain medications can trigger lupus; hormones since it is more prevalent in women, particularly those of childbearing age, hormonal factors are thought to play a role. The disease is accompanied by a variety of circulating antibodies, the best known of which is the antinuclear antibody (ANA).

3.4 Risk factors

Pregnancy itself does not constitute a risk to patients with SLE, and essentially, placentas and fetus are normal. However, fetal survival is reduced due to an increased number of abortions, maternal renal insufficiency, and preeclampsia, which is more frequently seen in patients with SLE [24–26]. Some antibodies of patients with SLE are transferred to the fetus, causing fetal growth restriction (FGR), congenital heart block, thrombocytopenia, leukopenia, hemolytic anemia, skin lesions, discoid lupus, and a variety of other conditions, including the LE phenomenon which disappear within 2–5 months after delivery. The constellation of congenital heart block with fetal hydrops and skin lesions is considered part of neonatal lupus syndrome. Several risk factors are associated with the development of LE such as gender (women are at a higher risk than men), and it is mostly diagnosed between ages 15 and 55; ethnicity. Family history, namely the presence of a relative with lupus or another autoimmune disease, increases risk; infections (viruses, bacteria, and protozoa) can trigger lupus or cause a flare-up. Several infections were revealed to cause immune dysfunction by molecular mimicry, epitope spreading, and bystander activation, and in contrast, certain pathogens were revealed to protect from immune dysregulation. Medications such as procainamide, hydralazine, and quinidine have been linked to drug-induced lupus.

3.5 Pathology

3.5.1 Gross placental findings

Although placentas may appear normal upon macroscopic examination, more often, they show changes virtually indistinguishable from lesions caused by preeclampsia, with the particularity that SLE changes typically occur in the second trimester. These findings include reduced size and weight, infarcts, thrombosis, necrosis, and retroplacental hematomas (see **Figure 1**).

3.5.2 Microscopic features

The placenta from an SLE-affected pregnancy most typically reveals alterations classifiable as maternal vascular malperfusion (MVM). These include villous changes such as atrophy, fibrosis, increased syncytial knots, and X-cell proliferation.

Inflammation, by chronic villitis with the presence of an intervillous lymphocytic and plasmocytic infiltrate, and decidual vasculopathy marked by the thickening and hyalinization of the walls of decidual blood vessels, frequently accompanied by fibrinoid necrosis. Furthermore, infarctions, areas of coagulative necrosis, and thrombotic lesions can also be present (see **Figure 2**). With that in mind, the presence of decidual vasculopathy and infarcts in the second trimester, whether in association with preeclampsia, or not, suggests the possibility of undiagnosed SLE.

4. Antiphospholipid syndrome and lupus anticoagulant

4.1 Definition

Antiphospholipid syndrome (APS) and Lupus anticoagulant are autoimmune disorders the first defined by the occurrence of venous and/or arterial thromboses and/or recurrent pregnancy morbidity in the presence of persistent positivity for antiphospholipid antibodies (aPL) [27]. Primary antiphospholipid syndrome is characterized by thrombosis and autoantibodies directed against phospholipids or associated proteins, but the genetic etiology of PAPS remains unknown [28]. Characterized by circulating autoantibodies best known for increased risk of multiple thromboses. Lupus anticoagulant (LA) is the most observed of several antiphospholipid antibodies. In pregnancy, antiphospholipid syndrome is referred to as obstetrical APS (OAPS), and it is associated with several complications such as preeclampsia, recurrent miscarriage, premature birth, and even fetal death [13, 26]. While the presence of these antibodies can be indicative of APS, their exact role and the factors contributing to it development are complex and multifaceted.

4.2 Demography

Female predominance, with a female/male ratio of 5/1. This predominance is even more pronounced in patients with systemic lupus erythematosus (SLE), where the female/male ratio increases to 7/1. In contrast, primary antiphospholipid syndrome (PAPS) exhibits a lower female/male ratio of 3.5/1 [28]. Between 2000 and 2015, 33 incident cases of APS were identified by the Sydney criteria in a cohort where the average age of the study population was 54.2 years, and 97% were Caucasian [29].

4.3 Etiology

APS is an autoimmune disease associated with systemic autoantibodies such as IgA isotypes, anticardiolipin antibodies (aCL), lupus anticoagulant (LA), and anti-β2-glycoprotein antibodies (anti-β2GPI) [29]. Genetics likely play a crucial role in increasing a person's risk of developing APS, although the specific genes involved are not yet fully understood. Guffroy et al. results provide evidence of genetic heterogeneity in PAPS, even in a homogeneous series of triple patients [30].

4.4 Risk factors

It is believed that genetic predisposition, combined with environmental and lifestyle factors, can significantly influence the likelihood of developing APS.

Understanding the interplay between genetics, lifestyle factors, and the presence of antiphospholipid antibodies is essential for managing and mitigating the risk of APS. While more research is needed to pinpoint the specific genetic factors involved [30], current knowledge highlights the importance of addressing modifiable risk factors such as smoking, hypertension, obesity, and the use of estrogen-containing medications. For individuals with antiphospholipid antibodies, being aware of these risk factors and taking proactive steps to manage them can significantly reduce the likelihood of developing blood clots and the associated complications of APS. It is possible for individuals to produce antibodies that attack phospholipids without developing blood clots or experiencing the clinical manifestations of APS. This indicates that the mere presence of antiphospholipid antibodies is not sufficient to cause the syndrome. Several other contributing factors are necessary to trigger the pathological processes leading to blood clot formation. For individuals with antiphospholipid antibodies, smoking, hypertension, obesity, and estrogen-containing medications further increase the likelihood of clot development by contributing to vascular injury, inflammation, increased blood viscosity, and reduced fibrinolytic activity, adding additional stress to the cardiovascular system promoting clot formation. For individuals with antiphospholipid antibodies, the presence of another autoimmune condition like lupus heightens the risk of thrombosis due to the compounded effects of inflammation and immune dysregulation. Also, women with histories of repeated abortion and premature births often possess circulating lupus anticoagulant (LA) antibodies that may indirectly be responsible for increased fetal wastage. LA positivity was found in 6% of pregnancy morbidity cases, 10% of deep vein thrombosis cases, 11% of myocardial infarction cases, and 14% of stroke cases [31, 32]. However, the literature is heterogeneous regarding the types of AL tests, definitions of positivity, and clinical manifestations [33].

4.5 Pathology

4.5.1 Gross placental findings

Gross placental findings reflect the hypercoagulable (thrombosis) state associated with APS. The main feature in these cases is that previous conditions are normally associated with large and numerous areas of infarction and necrosis (see **Figure 1**) due to interrupted blood flow, hemorrhage, and fibrotic tissue related to chronic vascular compromise.

4.5.2 Microscopic features

Are related to hypoxic and ischemic injury or high-speed blood flow that damages the placenta. This results in decreased or interrupted maternal blood flow to the placenta and a lack of nutrients for the fetus. Parenchymal lesions are associated with decidual vasculopathy characterized by thickened, fibrotic, and sometimes necrotic decidual vessels with fibrinoid deposits (see **Figure 2A**), villous changes related to villous trophoblastic damage and syncytial knots (see **Figure 2B**), indicating stress and hypoxia. Sometimes, vasculitis (inflammation of blood vessels), widespread thrombi within both maternal and fetal placental vessels, and chronic inflammation is present, particularly in the intervillous space and chorionic villi. Decreased number and size of blood vessels in the chorionic villi (villi reduced vascularity), leading to impaired nutrient and oxygen exchange, and infarctions (coagulative necrosis) within the placental parenchyma are other types of lesions.

5. Thrombophilia

5.1 Definition

Thrombophilia, also called hypercoagulability or prothrombotic condition, usually reflects a certain imbalance that occurs either in the coagulation cascade or in the anticoagulation/fibrinolytic system, platelets, and the vessel wall (Virchow's Triad). Usually categorized as inherited or acquired, it can lead to both venous and arterial clots. Thrombotic complications are associated with multiorgan failure (such as deep vein thrombosis (DVT), pulmonary embolism, and stroke). Inherited thrombophilia have an impact on human reproduction and increased mortality including fetal death. These emphasize the importance of diagnosing and initiating thromboprophylaxis. So, studies on the genetic profiles of proteins involved in thrombophilia and thrombotic events are of great importance, both in treating and in preventing deaths [34].

5.2 Demography

Thrombophilia affect individuals worldwide, but their prevalence can vary based on the type and population. Due to the multitude and complexity of inherited thrombophilia, the true prevalence is unknown, and current data may be providing an underestimate [35, 36]. Comparison among different epidemiologic studies becomes difficult due to variations in study design and inclusion criteria [35, 36].

Clinical diagnosis is based on medical history, physical examination, laboratory data, and imaging. Genetic testing is useful for confirming diagnosis, differential diagnosis, recurrence risk evaluation, and asymptomatic diagnosis in families with a known mutation. Differential diagnosis should consider the above conditions and secondary causes of thrombosis.

The prevalence of common inherited thrombophilia is variable among both healthy patients and patients with recurrent thrombosis. According to epidemiologic and modeling studies obtained from certain sources, the prevalence of inherited thrombophilia was estimated to be between 0.01 and 7% in Caucasians [35, 36]. In certain studies, the incidence of incident and recurrent venous thrombosis in inherited disorders is approximately 150–840 and 3500–10,500 per 100,000 individuals, respectively [36]. It may be a misdisorder, with an incident rate of 1 in 100,000 children, 1 in 1000 adults, and 1 in 100 elderly people worldwide each year [34–36].

5.3 Etiology

Thrombophilia may develop in patients irrespective of their age groups. Although acquired thrombophlias are more commonly observed among elderly patients who are more than 60 years old, inherited thrombophilia are more common in young patients between 40 and 55 years old [34, 35]. Inherited thrombophilia has autosomal dominant, autosomal recessive, or X-linked inheritance. This is related to deficiencies of natural anticoagulants (antithrombin, protein C, and protein S), increased homocysteine values, and changes in fibrinogen and coagulation factors. One important thing to note is that hereditary thrombophilia increases the risk of miscarriage. Acquired thrombophilia occurs as a result of secondary diseases, such as autoimmune disorders, trauma, or malignancy. The etiology of the most common inherited form is related to several mutations and factor Leiden deficiency mutations, leading to resistance to activate protein C [34]. Prothrombin G20210A mutation results in increased levels of prothrombin [34]. Protein C and Protein S deficiency increases clotting risk, and antithrombin III deficiency leads to an increased risk of thrombosis [34]. The more common acquired thrombophilia is antiphospholipid syndrome (APS), which is characterized by the presence of antiphospholipid antibodies that increase clotting risk [34]. Other conditions such as hyperhomocysteinemia, can damage blood vessel linings and increase clot risk [34]. Also certain cancers, prolonged immobility, and the use of hormone replacement therapy or oral contraceptives can increase thrombosis risk.

5.4 Risk factors

Several factors can increase the risk of developing thrombophilia such as genetics related to a family history of thrombophilia or increasing blood clots; race, the factor V Leiden G1691A and prothrombin G20210A mutations usually affect Caucasian individuals; age and gender, certain groups observed an increased risk of thrombosis in younger females and older males, while others found similar frequencies in both [35]. Pregnancy due to hormonal changes; surgery or trauma, prolonged immobility related to bed rest or long flights and lifestyle factors (smoking), obesity, and contraceptives or hormone replacement therapy are hypercoagulability and prothrombotic conditions that promote clot formation [34–36].

5.5 Pathology

5.5.1 Gross placental findings

In pregnancies affected by thrombophilia, the placenta may show several gross abnormalities like infarctions associated with areas of dead tissue due to lack of blood supply; Retroplacental (or intramural) hematomas corresponding a blood clot behind (or inside) the placenta and excessive fibrin deposition (a protein involved in clotting) on the placental surface are frequent (see **Figure 1**); like as a small or poorly developed placenta due to compromised blood flow.

5.5.2 Microscopic features

Microscopic features are characterized by thrombi in fetal vessels; decidual vasculopathy; infarcts hypertensive or usual type at different stages; increased fibrin deposition characterized by dense eosinophilic (pink-staining) material in parenchyma; fibrin thrombi in maternal space; and abnormalities of the chorionic villi (tiny finger-like projections that facilitate nutrient gas exchange). Understanding these features is crucial for diagnosing and managing thrombophilia, especially in the context of pregnancy, where the adverse risks to both mother and fetus can be significant.

6. Diabetes mellitus and gestational

6.1 Definition

Diabetes mellitus (DM) is a chronic metabolic disorder characterized by high blood glucose levels (hyperglycemia) due to defects in insulin secretion, insulin action, or both. The two main types are type 1 DM (T1D) and type 2 DM (T2D). The former is an autoimmune condition where the body's immune system attacks insulin-producing beta cells in the pancreas. Type 2 DM is characterized by insulin resistance and relative insulin deficiency often associated with obesity. Gestational diabetes mellitus (GDM) is a common pregnancy complication, and hyperglycemia in pregnancy (HIP) is described as the most common metabolic abnormality in pregnant women. It is spontaneous hyperglycemia, not clearly type 1 or type 2, developing during pregnancy, typically resolves after delivery but increases the risk of developing type 2 DM later in life [37]. In 2014, the World Health Organization (WHO) defined HIP as diabetes first detected at any time during pregnancy, along with pre-existing diabetes, and is further sub-classified as diabetes in pregnancy (DIP) and gestational diabetes mellitus (GDM) [38, 39].

6.2 Demography

According to the most recent (2019), International Diabetes Federation (IDF) showed a slight reduction in the overall HIP prevalence to 15.8%, with GDM at 12.8% and DIP at 2.6%, made up of hyperglycemia first detected in pregnancy and pre-existing diabetes both respectively at 1.3% [39].

GDM affects approximately 14% of pregnancies worldwide, representing approximately 18 million births annually [38]. However, recent factors such as differences in screening approaches and changes in diagnostic criteria have confounded the prevalence rates [38].

6.3 Risk factors

The risk factors for diabetes in pregnancy depend on the type of diabetes: Type 1 diabetes often occurs in children or young adults, but it can start at any age. Diabetes during pregnancy is more common in women who have a family member with T2D. Overweight women and women who have had GD before and twins or other multiples are more likely to have T2D and GD.

6.4 Pathology

6.4.1 Gross placental findings

Placentas from GDM pregnancy are bigger and heavier than placentas from normal pregnancies [40]. T1D and GDM have increased placental weight and volume of parenchymal (villi, fetal vessels and maternal space) tissue.

6.4.2 Microscopic features

Microscopic features are characterized by increased frequency of immature villi (delayed villous maturation), villous edema, and hyperplasia; increased number of capillaries (redundant capillary connections) in terminal villi, chorangiosis; a significant increase of vascular lesions associated with fibrinoid necrosis, and ischemia, defined by increased maturation, band Tenney–Parker changes or microscopic/macroscopic infarcts, increase fibrin thrombi, and thickening of the basement membrane in the placentas, and increased incidence of nucleated fetal red blood cells in women with GDM and pregestational diabetes [40].

7. Conclusions

Maternal vascular malperfusion is the diagnosis given to placentas with gross and microscopic evidence of ischemia based on abnormal maternal perfusion. It is a composite diagnosis requiring more than one feature of placental ischemia, each one of which has a differential diagnosis.

The placentas of such pregnancies show similar changes associated with increased incidence of thrombosis, including intervillous thrombi, intervillous fibrinoid deposition, abruption, and fetal thrombotic vasculopathy. The most common sequelae of MVM is fetal growth restriction. Other sequelae include preterm delivery and intrauterine fetal demise.

At the pathological examination, the presence of infarcts and abruption and the percentage of placental tissue involved should be noted. The location of the infarcts (central versus peripheral) and stage (early versus late) of the lesions should also be recorded. Representative sections of the lesions should be taken along with routine sections. Extra sections to evaluate decidual vessels are also advised.

If there is no history of hypertensive disease, preeclampsia, or other systemic disease associated with these findings, a workup for the disorders noted above must be suggested in the pathological placental report.

Both mothers and surviving infants in pregnancies complicated by MVM in the placenta are at risk for developing cardiovascular disease. The treatment of MVM is to treat the cause, if possible. Modulation of risk for recurrence includes optimization of maternal health with a focus on cardiovascular status, glucose tolerance, attention to pre-pregnancy body mass index (BMI), associated pregnancy weight gain, and renal function.

Conflict of interest

The authors declare no conflict of interest.

Author details

Rosete Nogueira[1,2]* and Filipe Soares Nogueira[3]

1 ICVS/3B's PT Government Associate Laboratory, Life and Health Sciences Research Institute (ICVS), School of Medicine, University of Minho, Campus de Gualtar, Portugal

2 Placental and Embryo and Fetal Pathology Laboratory, LAP, Unilabs, Portugal

3 Hospital Garcia de Orta, Portugal

*Address all correspondence to: rosete.nogueira@med.uminho.pt

IntechOpen

References

[1] Roberts DJ, Polizzano C. Atlas of Placental Pathology. United States: American Registry of Pathology; 2021

[2] Redline RW, Boyd T, Campbell V, et al. Maternal vascular underperfusion: Nosology and reproducibility of placental reaction patterns. Pediatric and Developmental Pathology. 2004;7:237-249

[3] Lemos D, Braga AC, Nogueira R. Nonlinear regression on growth curves for placental parameters in R. In: Pereira AI, Mendes A, Fernandes FP, Pacheco MF, Coelho JP, Lima J, editors. Optimization, Learning Algorithms and Applications. OL2A 2023. Communications in Computer and Information Science. Vol 1981. Cham: Springer; 2023. DOI: 10.1007/978-3-031-53025-8_39

[4] Stojanovska V, Zenclussen AC. Innate and adaptive immune responses in HELLP syndrome. Frontiers in Immunology. 2020;11:667. DOI: 10.3389/fimmu.2020.00667

[5] Nogueira R et al. Placental biometric parameters the usefulness of placental weight ratio and birth/placental weight ratio percentile curves for singleton gestations as a function of gestational age. Journal of Clinical & Anatomic Pathology. 2019;4(104):1-15

[6] American College of Obstetricians and Gynecologists; Task Force on Hypertension in Pregnancy. Hypertension in pregnancy. Report of the American College of Obstetricians and Gynecologists' task force on hypertension in pregnancy. Obstetrics and Gynecology. 2013;122:1122-1131

[7] Savitz DA, Danilack VA, Engel SM, et al. Descriptive epidemiology of chronic hypertension, gestational hypertension, and preeclampsia in New York state, 1995-2004. Maternal and Child Health Journal. 2014;18:829-838

[8] von Dadelszen P, Magee LA, Roberts JM. Subclassification of preeclampsia. Hypertension in Pregnancy. 2003;22(2):143-148. DOI: 10.1081/PRG-120021060

[9] Vest AR, Cho LS. Hypertension in pregnancy. Current Atherosclerosis Reports. 2014;16:395

[10] Seely EW, Ecker J. Chronic hypertension in pregnancy. Circulation. 2014;18:829-838

[11] Staff AC, Sibai BM. Prevalence of preeclampsia and eclampsia. In: Taylor RN, Roberts JM, Cunningham FG, editors. Chesley's Hypertensive Disorders in Pregnancy. Amsterdam: Academic Press; 2014

[12] Riise HKR, Sulo G, Tell GS, et al. Association between gestational hypertension and risk of cardiovascular disease among 617589 Norwegian women. Journal of the American Heart Association. 2018;7:e008337

[13] Shen M, Smith GN, Rodger M, et al. Comparison of risk factors and outcomes of gestational hypertension and preeclampsia. PLoS One. 2017;12:e0175914

[14] Sava RI, March KL, Pepine CJ. Hypertension in pregnancy: Taking cues from pathophysiology for clinical practice. Clinical Cardiology. 2018;41:220-227

[15] Burton GJ, Woods AW, Jauniaux E, et al. Rheological and physiological

consequences of conversion of maternal spiral arteries for uteroplacental blood flow during human pregnancy. Placenta. 2009;**30**:473-482

[16] Jauniaux E, Hempstock J, Greenwold N, Burton GJ. Trophoblastic oxidative stress in relation to temporal and regional differences in maternal placenta blood flow in normal and abnormal early pregnancies. The American Journal of Pathology. 2003;**162**:115-125

[17] LaMarca B, Cornelius DC, Harmon AC, et al. Identifying immune mechanisms mediating hypertension during preeclampsia. American Journal of Physiology. Regulatory, Integrative and Comparative Physiology. 2016;**311**:R1-R9

[18] Klatsky PC, Delaney SS, Caughey AB, et al. The role of the embryonic origin in preeclampsia: A comparison of autologous in vitro fertilization and ovum donor pregnancies. Obstetrics and Gynecology. 2010;**116**:1387-1392

[19] Yong HEJ, Murthi P, Brenneck SP, et al. Genetic approaches in preeclampsia. Methods in Molecular Biology. 2018;**1710**:53-72

[20] Stojanovska V, Zenclussen AC. Innate and Adaptive Immune Responses in HELLP Syndrome. Frontiers in Immunology. 15 Apr 2020;**11**:667. DOI: 10.3389/fimmu.2020.00667. PMID: 32351511; PMCID: PMC7174768

[21] Ameer MA, Chaudhry H, Mushtaq J, Khan OS, Babar M, Hashim T, et al. An overview of systemic lupus erythematosus (SLE) pathogenesis, classification, and management. Cureus. 2022;**14**(10):e30330. DOI: 10.7759/cureus.30330

[22] Castellanos Gutierrez AS, Figueras F, Morales-Prieto DM, Schleußner E, Espinosa G, Baños N.

Placental damage in pregnancies with systemic lupus erythematosus: A narrative review. Frontiers in Immunology. 2022;**13**:941586. DOI: 10.3389/fimmu.2022.941586

[23] Feldman CH, Hiraki LT, Liu J, Fischer MA, Solomon DH, Alarcón GS, et al. Epidemiology and sociodemographics of systemic lupus erythematosus and lupus nephritis among US adults with Medicaid coverage, 2000-2004. Arthritis and Rheumatism. 2013;**65**(3):753-763. DOI: 10.1002/art.37795

[24] Dalal DS, Patel KA, Patel MA. Systemic Lupus Erythematosus and Pregnancy: A Brief Review. The Journal of Obstetrics and Gynaecology of India. Apr 2019;**69**(2):104-109. DOI: 10.1007/s13224-019-01212-8. Epub 2019 Mar 12. PMID: 30956462; PMCID: PMC6430271

[25] Clark CA, Spitzer KA, Laskin CA, DeSouza R. Preterm deliveries in women with systemic lupus erythematosus. Journal of Rheumatology. 2005;**32**(9):1674-1677

[26] Smyth A, Oliveira GH, Lahr BD, Bailey KR, Norby SM, Garovic VD. A systematic review and meta-analysis of pregnancy outcomes in patients with systemic lupus erythematosus and lupus nephritis. Clinical Journal of the American Society of Nephrology. 2010;**5**(11):2060-2068. DOI: 10.2215/CJN.00240110

[27] Jung JY, Suh CH. Infection in systemic lupus erythematosus, similarities, and differences with lupus flare. The Korean Journal of Internal Medicine. 2017;**32**(3):429-438. DOI: 10.3904/kjim.2016.234. Epub 2017 Apr 28

[28] Bobircă A, Dumitrache A, Alexandru C, Florescu A, Ciobotaru G, Bobircă F, et al. Pathophysiology of placenta in antiphospholipid syndrome.

Physiologia. 2022;**2**:66-79. DOI: 10.3390/physiologia2030007

[29] Barinotti A, Radin M, Cecchi I, Foddai SG, Rubini E, Roccatello D, et al. Genetic factors in antiphospholipid syndrome: Preliminary experience with whole exome sequencing. International Journal of Molecular Sciences. 2020;**21**(24):9551. DOI: 10.3390/ijms21249551

[30] Guffroy A, Jacquel L, Seeleuthner Y, Paul N, Poindron V, Maurier F, et al. An immunogenomic exome landscape of triple positive primary antiphospholipid patients. Genes and Immunity. 2024;**25**(2):108-116. DOI: 10.1038/s41435-024-00255-w. Epub 2024 Jan 24. Erratum in: Genes Immun; 2024 Apr;25(2):176. DOI: 10.1038/s41435-024-00261-y

[31] Cervera R, Boffa MC, Khamashta MA, Hughes GR. The euro-phospholipid project: Epidemiology of the antiphospholipid syndrome in Europe. Lupus. 2009;**18**(10):889-893. DOI: 10.1177/0961203309106832

[32] Duarte-García A, Pham MM, Crowson CS, Amin S, Moder KG, Pruthi RK, et al. The epidemiology of antiphospholipid syndrome: A population-based study. Arthritis & Rhematology. 2019;**71**(9):1545-1552. DOI: 10.1002/art.40901. Epub 2019 Aug 1. Erratum in: Arthritis Rheumatol; 2020 Apr;72(4):597. DOI: 10.1002/art.41241

[33] Erkan D, Sciascia S, Bertolaccini ML, Cohen H. APS ACTION executive committee. Antiphospholipid syndrome Alliance for clinical trials and international networking (APS ACTION): 10-year update. Current Rheumatology Reports. 2021;**23**(6):45. DOI: 10.1007/s11926-021-01008-8. Erratum in: Curr Rheumatol Rep; 2021 Jun 23;23(7):48. DOI: 10.1007/s11926-021-01034-6

[34] Siriez R, Dogné JM, Gosselin R, Laloy J, Mullier F, Douxfils J. Comprehensive review of the impact of direct oral anticoagulants on thrombophilia diagnostic tests: Practical recommendations for the laboratory. International Journal of Laboratory Hematology. 2021;**43**(1):7-20. DOI: 10.1111/ijlh.13342. Epub 2020 Sep 18

[35] Stevens SM, Woller SC, Bauer KA, Kasthuri R, Cushman M, Streiff M, et al. Guidance for the evaluation and treatment of hereditary and acquired thrombophilia. Journal of Thrombosis and Thrombolysis. 2016;**41**(1):154-164. DOI: 10.1007/s11239-015-1316-1

[36] Cohoon KP, Heit JÁ. Inherited and secondary thrombophilia. Circulation. 2014;**129**(2):254-257. DOI: 10.1161/CIRCULATIONAHA.113.001943

[37] Plows JF, Stanley JL, Baker PN, Reynolds CM, Vickers MH. The pathophysiology of gestational diabetes mellitus. International Journal of Molecular Sciences. 2018;**19**(11):3342. DOI: 10.3390/ijms19113342. Published online 2018 Oct 26

[38] World Health Organization. Diagnostic criteria and classification of hyperglycaemia first detected in pregnancy: A World Health Organization guideline. Diabetes Research and Clinical Practice. 2014;**103**:341-363

[39] International Diabetes Federation. IDF Diabetes Atlas. 9th ed. Brussels, Belgium: International Diabetes Federation; 2019

[40] Huynh J, Dawson D, Roberts D, Bentley-Lewis R. A systematic review of placental pathology in maternal diabetes mellitus. Placenta. 2015;**36**(2):101-114. DOI: 10.1016/j.placenta.2014.11.021. Epub 2014 Dec 5